BODY FULL OF STARS

BODY FULL *of* STARS

Female Rage *and* My Passage into Motherhood

MOLLY CARO MAY

COUNTERPOINT
BERKELEY, CALIFORNIA

Body Full of Stars

Copyright © 2018 by Molly Caro May

ISBN: 978-1-61902-489-2

The Library of Congress Cataloging-in-Publication Data is available.

Jacket designed by Donna Cheng
Book designed by Wah-Ming Chang

COUNTERPOINT
2560 Ninth Street, Suite 318
Berkeley, CA 94710
www.counterpointpress.com

Printed in the United States of America
Distributed by Publishers Group West

10 9 8 7 6 5 4 3 2 1

For

Mare and Eula and our shared body

Caring for myself is not self-indulgence, it is self-preservation,
and that is an act of political warfare.

AUDRE LORDE

What we profoundly need are rituals that take into regard
the blood, the shock, the heat, the shit, the anguish, the glory,
the earnestness of the female body.

LOUISE ERDRICH

CONTENTS

~

BODY FULL OF STARS

~

The fracture appears. You fall to your knees and wonder: is it situational, historical, chemical, ancestral, physiological, mental? It may be all of these. It may be none. Is it just who I am? Well, it isn't you and it is you. It is an energy you are meeting. Maybe for the first time. Maybe for the thousandth time. But now in a new way. It has a message. It wants to tell you something important. The last thing you want to do is listen. You want out. Get me the hell out. And if you can't get out, you want it gone, exiled, extracted from your essence. However, that's the basic Physics 101 truth about energy. It cannot be destroyed. Yes, you are responsible for how you manage it. But you aren't necessarily it. You are in relationship with it. You start to hear it, ask questions of it, even love it. This can be hard. This can also be easy. Then you ask it to reroute. Please and thank you. You are in a process of birthing some part of yourself. Your whole life is a series of births. We only learn and relearn this by living it.

Labor

"I wonder what the wind is bringing," I say.

"Who knows?" he answers, and grabs my hand. We are walking a long slow walk in late April. Snow edges around tamped-down grass. Small green buds have begun to surface. The wind almost blows my straw hat away and the moon was full last night. I have told my midwife about how it has always affected my cycles, but she says first babies often come two weeks late.

We'll see.

Because it is five days before my due date and I can feel the new mother-me nearby. She speaks to me already. She will walk through the forest for hours with her newborn tucked against her breast. As years unfold, she will pass on some necessary truths: cross many borders, language matters, don't forget to talk to your own body. Maybe motherhood will give her a reason to become a great human.

We duck under some trees and I lurch back down the hill, one hand on my belly, one hand on Chris's shoulder. A few weeks ago, at my yearly haircut, the same two-inch trim because I've never adventured much with my brown locks or my physical presentation, I told my tattooed hairdresser that my husband had started to go gray, a remarkable even blend with his dark, and she said, "Well, what you've got on your hands now is a salt-and-pepper fox."

And she's right, only, he is, of course, more than that.

We've been together for thirteen years and, despite our recent murky distance, he still does it for me on all levels.

When we reach flat ground, a great blue whale urge to rest comes over me. I curl up on the bed. Chris stays outdoors in the wintery mix of spring and rearranges rocks from our garden into a pile for a different garden. I've canceled all my plans for the next few days. My friends near and far know I've entered what I call the cave. My mother walks in from her house next door to where we are living, in her guesthouse, and smiles at me. We are all waiting.

"How are you, sweetheart?" she asks.

"Good, slow, ready. But this babe might wait until May."

"We'll see," she says. "I'm making a smoothie, would you like some?"

"Sure," I say, "thanks," and I watch my graceful mother walk out the door. She lived across the globe, away from her community, when she gave birth to me. As afternoon sun streaks through the window, I scroll through boy names on the phone. Hard to find one we like. We never had an ultrasound but my intuition knows this babe is a boy. We may never get to use the girl name we chose. I glance out the window and whisper it aloud anyway. Then my bladder calls out.

It's hard to remember what it felt like to inhabit a non-pregnant body. I barrel-roll off the bed and stand up. Pop. Water starts to spill from between my legs. It is clear but pale green. I freeze, as if any more movement will cause a baby to drop from between my legs. Drums pound in my chest. What do I do now? My mother walks back in with my tiger dog Bru.

"I think my water just broke," I stutter.

"Looks like it," she says, and for a moment we look down, then a long pause, even Bru investigates. She has told me what her mother told her. My body will know what to do. It is a natural process. I've spent most my life in an intense conversation with my body—this will be one more part of that.

Water broke.

Water broke.

Water broken.

What does that even mean?

We stare as it pools on the concrete floor.

~

I come from brothers—so do my mother, my father, my husband, his mother, and his father. We have only brothers. There are no sisters and no girls, other than the ones who brought the boys into the world. I didn't care about the sex of my baby. Even so I dreamt of my son riding in a lime-green backpack, and of losing him, leaving him somewhere, and the panic. Did he know what a crazy lady his mother had become while he was in utero? At six weeks pregnant, I had perched on a chair in the office of my doctor and friend Holcomb.

"How do you feel—any nausea?" she asked.

"Not a bit. I feel great, excited," I beamed as my hand fluttered over a flat belly. My mother had only one whiff of nausea during her three pregnancies, so the forecast looked good for me. The next week, though, my stomach turned. I began to vomit into toilets, mason jars while driving, bushes behind the hardware store, kitchen bowls, snow, and my own lap. Multiple times a day. None of this is unusual. But it didn't go away after the first trimester. It tapered but stayed my whole pregnancy. My baby was grown on chicken, whole milk yogurt, and oatmeal. I ate nothing green. I took no prenatal vitamins. I pressed my face into grass to get away from offending smells: toast, coffee, forest fires. Holcomb was also pregnant, a month behind me. Her nausea never shifted into vomiting. She explained she had to hold it down, just *could not* let that lid off.

But my lid had blown off.

Part of me knew it was an initiation—to what though, I wasn't sure yet.

Even daily body maintenance became impossible. I stopped brushing my hair or wearing sunscreen. Someone told me metal near my body was bad, so I cut one underwire out of my bra, forgot about the other, and walked around with uneven breasts for months without realizing it. My exuberance about life would kick in from time to time. I'd always been able to get up and try again. But then

7

something would backfire, like moving too fast too wide and long on cross-country skis and ending up at a chiropractor's office with seized muscles and ligaments around my pelvis.

It was a mild case of hyperemesis.

That would have been the rational explanation. But, being a constant believer in the metaphysical, I wondered, as usual, if my soul had created this situation *for* me. My closest friends knew me well enough to preempt me and say, "This is not your fault; you did not create this." Acid in my throat must be an act of releasing the old. It was necessary for my growth, right? I could also no longer censor what words came out of my mouth, except when teaching writing workshops in town. Somehow my sickness never showed up in front of my adult students or clients. Maybe I could control it then because I had control there. Chris and I had entered a cohabitation of sorts with my parents two months into my pregnancy when they moved permanently to their small cabin on this wild stretch of land in Montana. We had made a home here for two years in our own yurt until the cold and throwing up off the porch in the middle of the night got difficult. I needed the bathroom of the cabin. Their guesthouse was a garage, not yet a guesthouse. I wanted to welcome them to *their* land and then leave to rent a place nearby. But we couldn't both rent and save for the future home Chris would start to build soon on a triangle of land a thousand feet down the driveway. No bank would give a loan to a self-employed artist couple. My parents had been generous in letting us stay.

But the close quarters grated on everyone, especially me.

We slept on their couches, folding up and stashing blankets every morning. We shared the one small bathroom. Intergenerational. People used to live this way. Many still do. It could be a healthy support system. It could also be thunderstorms after thunderstorms. It was probably both.

A viper awoke in me.

Call it rage. Call it fury.

I wasn't unfamiliar with the emotion. It's a part of every human, but never before had it come on in and taken over. Everyone safe enough to be close annoyed me. I lashed out with mean comments. I apologized as much as I vomited. They watched me scream at the

moon. They backed away slowly. Chris and I happened to simultane-
ously be in the middle of an uncomfortable changing of the tides. We
avoided each other or stewed. No one saw me whack the ground re-
peatedly with a long metal spoon. Friends told me to feel the feelings.
C'mon, now. But my rage turned inward as well. How could I be so
cruel to the people supporting me? I'd never been a placid human,
always slightly impatient, but these maneuvers were new. I was losing
opportunities all over the place. My disappointment at not being a
radiant pregnant woman was a small part of it. My mother would
later say, "You were radiant at times. You just couldn't see it." She
would remind me there has always been a good and kind Molly and
point out I had lost control of some basics all at once—my shelter, my
adulthood, my marriage, my mode of transportation, and my body.
There *are* photos of me with my arms around Chris, with a wide smile
and gleam in my eyes, with my hands wrapped around the gorgeous
largess of my body. Toward the end, a softening occurred. It has to
when all you can do is waddle. I would stand on a snowy bridge, tap
my belly, and feel a small kick respond back.

"Hey there, sweets."

My babe was already my purifier.

My body, despite the throwing up, had stayed strong through the
pregnancy—no swollen ankles, no blood pressure spike, no low iron,
no infections, no complications at all. I held on to this luck. It was
my ticket back to decency. I had clawed my way through a strange
passage toward motherhood. Part of me destroyed by it; part of me
fortified. On the other end, we would meet our dear child, eventually
move into our house, and my body would no longer be stuck in a state
of shock. With that, I would let go of all rage and settle back into the
woman I knew myself to be.

It was my, our, backstory.

It's hard to erase the backstory.

~

The white stucco wall talks to me. *Dear, dear, Molly, hello.* It has white
on white shapes. I know it knows I know everything will be fine. My

9

knees tuck up into a fetus position as the fetus inside me feels the squeeze of these contractions. Three almond butter crackers sit on the ledge, lined up and ready to be sustenance later. Someone taught me a three-count breath. It becomes a rock shelter in the ocean. I go there. I rest there. Chris rubs me when I call to him. My midwife drifts through the front door and unbuttons her orange wool wrap with gusto. That might be last time my eyes open. She rubs my lower back. Her hand is cool and I don't want her to stop. She checks my cervix. I am six centimeters dilated, good work for the already nine hours of labor through the night. But I am missing something. I am missing something important. What is it? Fear. I can't find my fear. It's usually so loud, but it isn't here. I peer into dark corners for it. Maybe it is hiding.

Did it take anger with it too?

Someone catches my vomit in a metal bowl.

"I know how to vomit," I say aloud, and laugh between heaves. It is nothing. It is easy to vomit. My midwife tells me that means we are close to transition. When I step into the tub, she warns me water can slow labor. But it doesn't. I keep on trucking. This is what the women in my family do. My knees touch bottom. I drape arms over the edge and sway my body. Another midwife arrives. Hipbones are opening. I feel them parting, making space.

"I can see your hips opening," Chris says from behind me.

What kind of animal am I? I am many animals. My lips are loose. Deep moans. Those are mine. "Good, stay low tone," my midwife says, and then, when my tone crescendos up, she reminds me, low, low, low. I do know how to let go of control. These animals tell me so. They are telling me something about who the child inside me will be. They are also telling me to push.

My body knows what to do.

"Reach down and feel the head," my midwife says.

"Nothing," I say. There is nothing.

She feels between my legs and then asks me to sit up. I don't want to.

"I sure would love to hear that baby's heart rate," she says, and then I am pulled out of the water and, after a few new positions, someone is putting a too-tight T-shirt on me. The sky outside blinds me until I am lying in the back of a van as it drives fast toward the hospital. It isn't an emergency, they tell me. I look for my fear but it has fled the scene completely. Chris holds my head. My midwife straddles me and holds an oxygen mask to my face. She asks me not to push—over and over.

"Don't push, don't push, try not to push."

I don't understand. I don't understand how to do that. The waves. So many waves—they won't stop, they can't. Does she know she is asking me to stop the ocean? The other midwife, driving, tells me to breathe out in fast short breaths. The animal in me reminds me that all of this, except the van zooming and banking corners on country roads, is ancient. I start to map the route in my mind. We are at this turn. There's that turn. We are close. Once we get there, it will all be over.

"I know you didn't plan to be here," the doctor says as nurses help me onto my back and my eyes close again. Nothing changes. We are only here because they can monitor better at the hospital. For five hours, I push. I'm sure it's been forty years of pushing. Someone get my baby out of me. Are casual conversations actually happening around me? What are they discussing? The nurses are ready to wheel me to the operating room. I don't know any of this. The doctor bends toward me and asks if he can use the vacuum. I gaze up at my midwife. She is surrounded by a halo of fluorescent light.

"It's a good option at this stage," she says, measuring out her words. So I say yes and close my eyes.

He puts the plunger in me.

Now *this* is pain. Fire before the actual fire of my child emerging. Yell, yell, yell, and I tell everyone I'm so tired.

"Open your eyes," Chris whispers to me, and he looks right into me, familiar eyes, love eyes. "You are strong. You are doing this."

I close my eyes again. I don't hear the machines beeping or the sound of my baby's heart rate dipping down, dangerous and low.

"Open your eyes," the doctor says on the second set of pushes with the plunger.

"Open your eyes," says my midwife.

"Look at me," the doctor says.

I look.

"You have to push your baby out *now*," he says.

And the mother bear in me wakes up, shakes out her fur, and roars.

My daughter comes out pink with her fist at her head, raised like a warrior. She comes from between my legs, moves toward my chest, leans toward me, stares right at me, our first gaze, eye to eye. In that stare, she says, *Hello,* and also, *Here we go.*

"Hey," I say.

"I am never doing that again," follows soon after, but I want to immediately disown my words because they aren't true. My whole body twitches with the betrayal of my language. I am just playing some part from a film. Chris is missing out. He'll never get the chance to be a laboring woman connected to earth and sky and animal and heat and dark and light and nothingness. She is the woman I will go on the search for during the messy after that is to come. She knows herself. She knows her body is a planet. I could drop and do one hundred push-ups. I. Am. A. Star. I gaze down at my daughter. Does she miss my womb, how it hugged her and encouraged her to go, go, go meet the world? She looks like my husband's brother. Maybe that is what I sensed when I sensed boy.

Her face, oh, her everything face.

"That was awesome," one of the nurses says, and she points to her armpits to show me the sweat on her scrubs. "*You* were awesome."

The doctors expected a blue baby, a non-breathing baby. Later, my midwife will explain I would have eventually pushed her out without the vacuum but she may have suffered oxygen deprivation. Each push compressed the umbilical cord wrapped around her body, cutting off her source of blood and oxygen. Her fist-and-head combo also made her "a very hard package" to deliver.

Fear sees me, watches me from the corner of a room bustling with nurses. It's back. I don't want it back. It asks me how I am going to raise a girl to love herself or her body. How will she be safe? How will she ever see her own beauty? It goads me, pokes at me with an iron stick.

~

The part of the story I will continue to forget is what happens right after birth. The placenta slides out—purple and dense and all-radiant sea creature. My doctor announces only one tiny perineal tear. May not even need a stitch.

Oh good. Oh phew.

Oh, wait. They are all staring at my vagina. Wait a minute. He sees something else. He has to investigate deep. Ow. Enough. It's over. Let me be. But there is a gash from my cervix to vaginal opening, probably from her elbow. They call for a surgeon. My daughter and Chris are taken outside so the anesthesiologist has the privacy required by law to give me a one-minute spinal tap injection. I want my babe in my arms. Everyone is safe, everyone is safe, we are safe, though. They numb my body after a non-numb birth. The surgeon pulls scrubs over her jeans and flowered shirt. She tells me she will have to spread me *wide* open to get in there. I watch her focus. "Is this your last surgery of the day?" I want to ask but don't. I am grateful a woman is the one sewing my womanhood back together. Still I will forget this scene over and over again. I don't know why we remember what we remember and why we forget what we forget.

~

What I learn: My female parts connect me to all other women. This is obvious and not so obvious. I get to choose what to do with those parts and how exactly to be what we call *female*. But they have a history beyond my own. Though we are finally now starting to recognize the gender binary as false, it has raised me. I cannot separate my female parts from the way my culture has oriented or disoriented me. I happen to identify with the gender ascribed to my anatomy. Female, though, is different than feminine. Everyone has some dosage of feminine energy, but it would seem that only a woman's body has an inherent femaleness. I'm talking pure biology here. A woman's pelvis looks like an alabaster fan with holes reaching up to the sky. Within the bone structure, layers of pink muscles, fascia, and ligaments cross over one another in an elaborate web of support we call the pelvic floor. It would be more accurate to call it a bowl, shaped much like a hammock. When we leap, walk, and move around, it holds up the uterus, bladder, and rectum—does the same in the male body. The pelvic bowl also supports the most essential part of a woman's potential. The organ of her womb functions as a creative center far beyond growing a child. Our ideas and intuition originate here. It is a portal. It has a pulse. It is here a woman can converse with ancestors, herself, and any energy that shows up.

~

The white sun. The cottonwood leaves. I stand in the dirt driveway and squint up at them. Bru moves his wet nose up and down my legs. He had heard me laboring and then smelled blood. Probably thought I died. For now, my non-mother self is gone. The empowerment of birth has postured me—straight back, proud, a woman who also recognizes not all women, sadly, get to feel this way. This new mother-me appeared. She's still on the astral plane. She's changing diapers like a pro. She is ready to sacrifice. I bend down so he can smell the swaddled package of my daughter. My daughter. Our daughter. We are bringing her home from the hospital. Nothing has ever been so complete. Once inside, I ease myself onto the inflatable orange donut on the rattan rocking chair of my childhood. This isn't easy. I almost slide off. There is a deep painful throb in my vagina. My shirt, well, it's a thin muslin navy button-down with tiny cream flecks. I wore it much of my pregnancy and will wear it almost every day for the next few months. Eventually, I will cut it up and make a handkerchief for my daughter. It makes me feel like I am wearing a sky of stars. "Here, Mom, hold her," I say, and I hand my black-haired daughter to my mother, who will be called Mare. Someone takes a photo of this moment—Mare holding her granddaughter up, while I lean over to gaze down at my daughter as my mother looks up at me, her daughter, now a mother of a daughter. Maybe we inherit the way we move through a passage. Maybe we inherit our assumptions. It is this matrilineal lineage I want to tell my daughter about. It is this matrilineal lineage I want to tell myself about.

~

My life begins with my mother. Under the red spread of a southwestern desert, she sat with graduate school friends in the bubbling waters of a hot tub. My father tumbled toward her, away from the non-clutch of his family. He chose to study the business of internationals because he had been raised as an international. My mother chose to study it because she, from Illinois, was not an international and thought it might be good to be. She had grown up in a place of neighbors, ice-skating, massive oak trees, and a malt shop. Her mother, Patricia, my Pat-Pat, an unfulfilled woman of study and intellect, had once told her: "Well, at least your hair isn't completely straight, at least you have a *bend* in it." But now here was my mother—in a navy blue bikini, her blue eyes framed by a pleat of dark straight hair. He later offered to fix her bicycle. When he crouched in the foyer, fiddling with a wrench and tire pump, my mother answered the phone call of another suitor while opening the front door to a bouquet of flowers from yet another. She had been a makeup model in Japan in her early twenties. One day, the large Helena Rubinstein poster of her would grace our living rooms in many countries. She was shy, though, a good Catholic girl. My father was a mannered mystery to her.

She wrote a letter to her parents to tell them some of her friends thought this new boyfriend of hers looked like Omar Sharif. Was he "an Arab"? her midwestern father wondered back in a letter. He was as white American as she was, but the dust of other places had settled on him, shined him up so he glittered something different.

When my mother's parents finally met him, Pat-Pat, in an unprecedented move, stood up for her by saying, "I think Mary is fond of this young man." Their union took them to a city, where they lived in an apartment with water dripping from the ceiling. On their first night, my mother cried when her new husband brought her an old shrimp salad sandwich from a deli. They both worked, and my mother walked the pavement as a salesperson for IBM.

They moved across the largest ocean.

They began their life as internationals.

She walked the foreign pavement of Australia for a new sales job. On her free days, she strolled down to the market to meet ocean air and eat fresh peaches and plums. I was conceived and her belly grew round. On that wharf, she wore silk scarves in her hair and ran her hand over her middle. She was sure the child inside her was a boy. The pregnancy was easy. Not much changed. She folded laundry with the same elegance she arranged vegetables on a cutting board. Every member of her family lived nine thousand miles away. But she would have never called herself alone. She wasn't that type.

Her labor was long.

I don't know whether she was lonely.

I suspect she sunk into the process and didn't dwell.

It ended with forceps, for the girl within her was not yet ready to emerge, a pattern that would repeat years later when that girl brought forth her own. Neither one of us ever expected to become a mother to a daughter. My mother's motherhood, as common as ether, began in that stark hospital room.

From your body I come, from my body I come.

~

My mother was told to put me on my stomach. I slept on my back. These days everyone says to put "the baby" on her back. My daughter wants her stomach. She sleeps on her side and we face each other nose to nose. Sometimes she trumpets like an elephant. I am awake always, listening. When I doze in the twilight, the weight of my arm over her body produces a satisfied sigh from her. She also likes to push her arms out between us. I know so little about what she likes or doesn't like yet. Except that she likes my hair. I usually wear it up in a loose bun because the humid climates of my childhood turned curls to frizz. The dry West does good things for it. But now, now I wear it down—messy, female, dark, curly. It's gorgeous to me now. Maybe it's the hormones. I don't ever want to put it up. I don't ever want to put real clothes on. I haven't gone anywhere. I don't know how long we've been here in the cave. People say a baby can come between a man and woman, but it's the opposite for us—he and his dark eyelashes, the way he cradles our baby, is perfection to me. It no longer matters that I was so sick during pregnancy. My irritation with him has vanished. We sit on the gray flannel chairs nursing. Her little mouth suckles. Her eyes pause at one of my long brown curls, like she's trying to place it, understand it. Does she reach for it? What is *that*? My curl becomes the first world-based pattern she notices. It spirals down to almost touch her. She will have curls of her own soon.

~

My new job is manager of bowel movements. When my newborn, my dog, and I all poop before 10 a.m., it's a good day and the goodness of it morphs me into a super-accomplished woman. I can't seem to clean or cook anything. My mom brings us food every day. She walks through the wooden door with plates of green beans, frittata, chicken Milanese, piles of arugula, turkey chili, yellow rice, elk stew. This is what she does. This is what she has always done with food. I don't know what women do alone, or why it makes any sense to not have others to help tend during this time.

"Do you have a name yet?" my mother asks with a coy smile as she arranges a plate and fork on the pillow next to my girl. Not yet. She is almost a week old. What *is* her name? Is it the one we originally thought of? We wanted to wait to know her. She looks like her uncle and grandfathers, in equal measure. It's a cliché that first children resemble the father, part of nature's DNA test. My mother used to playfully call me Kenitha because my face was so much like my father, Ken. Now family friends exclaim how much I am my mother. But I'm interested in giving her a name that will match her essence.

Chris leaves our cave for a few hours to find a rock for her naming. We are ceremony people. My body hums as I wait. He returns with two white creek stones: one for her, one for her parents. We had made a cairn with them, and the savage wind of last week scattered them to the ground. We place one next to our sleeping child. At the end of my pregnancy, Chris saw the name on a *Harper's Magazine* cover. The name comes from the Spanish patron saint of peace and speech and the Scandinavian word for sea gem. My childhood Spain. His ancestral Sweden. We don't know yet it is also an old, common name in the American South. It's unusual and old at the same time. In its Greek origin point, the name means *well spoken*. Well spoken. That matters to me. If there is one message I want to pass to my daughter, it is to speak her own truth.

Your language matters, my love.

We call my parents into the guesthouse and tell them.

Eula.

E-U-L-A, I spell it for them.

"Oh," my mom sighs. "Like *eulogy*."

My father tries to recover for her, for them.

They will like, even love it, in a few weeks, but it shocks them now, as it will shock Chris's family too. His parents will respond with silence. My brothers will be the only ones who honor it through the phone lines.

I try not to spit out my response.

"Did you really expect something like *Sarah* from us? You should be happy we didn't name her Sagebrush."

"What were your other options?" my mom asks.

Chris shoots a look to me across the bed: *Don't you dare tell her; don't you dare give away your power on this one.* The trees out the window sway and shake. I swear I hear sandhill cranes croaking nearby. I don't even know what time of year it is anymore.

"I'm not telling you," I say, and hold Eula closer to my breast.

~

It's been almost a month. No stretch marks. Not one. My mother didn't have any either. My stomach seems back to normal, with a little extra softness. Am I even thinner than before? I can eat vegetables again. My nipples are cracked but an herbal balm helps. The bleeding hasn't fully stopped. During my first walk on gravel and grass down to the mailbox, my pad overflows with what I assume is lochia, that watery post-birth fluid. "Maybe it's a ton of cervical fluid," I laugh to

Chris. I've been charting my menses for years now, sorting out what tacky versus creamy versus egg-white means for my health and my fertility. But, of course, it can't be cervical fluid—not in that quantity. My midwife thinks it's probably urine. Am I that out of it not to notice urine? Don't worry, she says. Do some Kegels. I can see a specialist, if necessary.

In general, I am pleased with my body.

Naked always, because there is no other way to be.

I move across the cold concrete floor to the bathroom like a woman in a trance. We don't sleep much, but I knew to expect that. The closest I get to being clothed is black cotton underwear. I've told everyone, including my father, to get used to my exposed breasts. The curtain of life has been pulled back now, so I am stripped down too. Somehow this exposure warrants me an openness with my parents that later will embarrass me. It will be exposure without really exposing myself. I stand in the doorjamb and explain my need to have a conversation with them individually about my beauty/body issues from childhood, how, once puberty hit, my appearance, and talk about it, started to exist in the negative space. "Oh, those May children are good-looking" became "Oh, those May boys are so handsome." I fell off the beauty map and stopped being included in that descriptor.

I became a pretty person who had gone off, like a pear does.

The grass blades outside smell of spring rain, and my newfound motherhood makes me urgent to evolve, let go, be better. They sip cans of lime-flavored LaCroix sparkling water and agree. They are always agreeable with me. I am ready to let go and forgive and ask for forgiveness, I say. My request is a demand. For the first time in my life, I want to tell them everything.

~

On our most recent visit to the midwives, one of them gets direct.

"You need to start wearing normal clothes again," she says to me.

"But they are in the basement, I don't know where they are, somewhere in duffel bags, I have no drawers to put them in," I respond, sheepish, and stare down at my Eula nuzzled against my too-small blue striped button-down. Are these also worn-out black yoga pants? Yes, they are.

"You need to go down to the basement and get them."

I'm shocked and a little shamed by this command. But I make myself understand she wants me to care for myself because caring for myself means caring for my baby. I get it. Eula, of course, is fine. She's gained the right amount of weight. She latches to the breast well. Nursing is easy. It doesn't hurt anymore. I realize this is lucky for us. So far, all goes well. I'm a little tired. Got to gather my clothing. Look forward to not wearing a pad to catch the postpartum blood. Look forward to getting to know my daughter.

But we are good.

I didn't burst into tears when my milk came in.

I haven't felt any postpartum blues.

I feel supported.

This helps me be attentive.

I sleep and heal when Chris wraps Eula against him and takes her on walks through the woods, up and down hills and under trees and a cloudy May sky, sounds of birds and water. I am tired but it is a clean and purposeful tired.

I am doing well.

We are doing well.

When we get home, I stomp into the kitchen and decide I don't want to put clothes on ever again, especially now that people want me to. Somewhere in the distance, I start to hear a sound, a whisper telling me that labor comes before labor and labor doesn't stop after labor. No one tells you really, the labor doesn't stop.

~

It's a text from Holcomb. During our pregnancies, we hiked together and talked about how much boy energy we both felt emanating from our uteruses. What would it be like to be in her body? So fit. So blond. So considered stunning by everyone. She's been waiting for her little one. And so *she* has come.

She.

Another girl.

"A girl," I whisper to Chris.

We both smile.

Fast small buzzes move like a current waking up within me. We have girls. We can do that girl thing together. They will learn to run fast and climb trees and be strong but also sensitive. They will have menses. We can welcome this moon cycle with love and openness. We can use the word *vagina* or *clitoris* with them. It suddenly feels so good to have a *we* in this. I don't have that with anyone else yet. I don't have a close friend with a girl who is the age of my girl. We can dive into ponds with our little women and teach them to love their bodies. These thoughts snowball as I pace around the house, as I do a little dance, and the snowball grows large and sparkly and powerful until it suddenly crashes.

What if her daughter is more beautiful than mine?

That's an awful thing to think when a baby is born, I tell myself. Who thinks that? No one wants to admit they think that. Stop it. And then sadness rushes through me. I am already worrying about Eula and how she will measure her own beauty. I recognize the projection. This is not something I want to pass on. Stop it, I tell myself, and I walk outside to sip some clear sweet mountain ether.

All. Is. Well. Everything. Is. Perfect.

Change a diaper.

Swaddle.

Eat zucchini.

Fold tiny pants.

~

It's my first day solo with my four-week-old daughter. Chris is going back to work—furniture to make, commissions to complete. Soon he will start to build our house, a one-man job. Goodbye, I'll see you in eight hours. He pulls on his old work pants, squeezes us both, and walks out the door.

Fear wakes up, stretches long wings, and flaps around in my chest cavity.

Please go away.

"We're okay, we're okay here," I say to us, and walk from bed to chair to dresser to kitchen and around again. In his absence, I become incapable of taking care of Eula, or myself. How will I eat? How will I shower? The gentle black ceiling fan now cuts the stale air. Unlike other new mothers, I can never put my daughter in the wrap. She doesn't like being in it with me, even when I offer the boob, because I can't bounce. Bouncing makes my vagina "fall out"—and pee, lots of pee, oceans of urine. If I put her down, she screams a baby dinosaur scream I can't handle yet. There is no way for me to be with her and have my hands free.

Now that we are alone, I need free hands.

"Please let's make this work," I whisper. I frog her legs and start to wrap her to me.

She wails and keeps the wails loud. I try to bounce her. I try to bounce her and a sort of hell breaks loose. Bru, now neglected, noses an empty water bowl I cannot bend down to fill, and as I bounce, pee soaks through my pad and through my unwashed yoga pants so that a puddle starts to form on the concrete floor and he, still thirsty, actually considers drinking that.

And Eula still screams.

One day this will be funny. Maybe.

Today, however, grief sprouts. I didn't want to be this kind of mother.

"Eula, stop, sweets, please stop," I beg her, my lips grazing her face.

Bru stares up at me.

When I call Chris, hours have passed.

He walks in and starts to set things right, unbothered that he had to leave work. He takes Eula. I mop up the mess. I might be crying a little about my failure, crying tears into my own pee, so many fluids. When I glance up, Chris is organizing the mess of everything everywhere as Eula snoozes wrapped against his calm chest, her little mouth open with the relief of it. He puts a gentle hand on my shoulder. A friend with a toddler told me not to worry if I freak out. Everyone freaks out. I plan not to let it happen again.

"I've got to go back," he says after some time.

"Okay, let's try to transfer her."

But as we are mid-transfer to my chest, I remember I forgot—somehow, god—to discard my urine-soaked pad and replace it with a fresh one. Eula must sense this as I secure the wrap. She wakes up. She goes from a quiet sea otter to a trapped and angry bat and I'm halfway to the bathroom, asking Chris to follow, to please change my pad for me. I am determined not to have to hand her over. I can do this. Surrounded by clean white tiles, I hold Eula in my wrap, trying to bounce her with my hands so I don't pee all over Chris's hands. He pulls my underwear down as I crouch over the toilet and try to tune out the crying. But when he opens the crinkly *Always* Extra-Long Pad with Wings, his know-how stops.

"I don't know how to put it on," he says.

"Just figure it out," I snap at this kind man who is just trying to help, who is doing something many men might not do, who I've come, over the years, to expect will accept the grit of body fluids with me without complaint or comment, and then "I'm sorry, I'm sorry," and his "It's okay, it's okay," and by the end of it, I can't tell who is or isn't crying anymore.

~

Friends call and I recount the birth like a wanderer returned from a long voyage. Traumatic, they ask, to be transferred to the hospital that way? No, no, no, just dramatic. I ride on the wild capacity of all women. Women *do* this. Women do this every day. Why don't we remind ourselves of that fact every day? We just move on because our bodies do what our bodies do.

Some days I am a master of the swaddle, of life.

Other days I am a failure of the swaddle, of life.

When Eula nurses, the light turns buttery. New grass shoots have pushed out of the earth. Snow melts. The importance of seasons has never been lost to me. I couldn't live somewhere where nature wasn't a constant presence, a reminder—this too, this everything you feel, it is a moment, it will shift, both what feels good and what feels bad. Her eyes flutter open and trace shadowy patterns and she unfolds, second by second, into everything I didn't expect.

No one in my birth class has looked at their vaginas yet. No one in my mother's nonexistent birth class would have looked either. Even my midwife gave me a friendly head nod and told me to hold off on investigating. I don't understand this. It took me so long to become a woman who actually looked; I can't stop now.

"Can you look for me?" I ask Chris because to squat over a mirror isn't possible yet.

I lay spread-eagle on the bed and hold myself open. He stands over me—one arm cradles our daughter, the other wields a spray bottle of water and lavender essential oil for healing. I've asked him to hose me down. I won't hide any of this gore from him. I want him to see the place his daughter came from. I know he is willing because he has always been up for anything and that was part of my draw toward him. I choose to trust that he'll be able to make the transition from *this is the birthing vagina* back to *this is the vagina I want to love on.*

"How does it look?" I ask.

"Um," he pauses, squints. "Great, babe," he says, "great." I know he is saying so simply because it is the right thing to say.

When I do look, the landscape has changed. Somehow this used to be there, but now it's somewhere else and where did that go, and what, what, oh god, is that? My midwife reorients me to my anatomy. Oh, okay. She'll find the vulva book so I can see all the vulvas out there in the world. There is a vulva book? How did I not know? I've never seen anyone's vulva but my own. Even the language; it is a vulva, not a vagina. The vagina is inside and, in Latin, means "sword holder." The vulva is outside, everything, the whole package. I know this. I knew this. But I had gone mainstream and called it vagina.

I don't remember my parents calling mine anything other than my "bottom."

I don't remember them talking about it at all.

I don't remember anyone around me mentioning it as a part of the body.

~

My mother walks in one morning and sits down on the rattan rocking chair. I've started to bleed again, big red stripes of blood. Not my menses, more postpartum blood. I've become skilled at disassociating from my body even when I don't think I am, so I don't mention the blood. I plan to will myself toward goodness and tell my mother Eula smiled today, five times. Before I speak, she asks if we've thought about where we will put the luggage in our new house.

Luggage. That is what matters right now? I don't want luggage. I don't want storage. I don't know why her comment bothers me so much.

"I don't know, Mom," I say to end the conversation.

She leaves.

Later, a friend will explain it to me: these moods are normal for a woman who has just gone through the hugest endurance event of anyone's life and a massive hormonal shift while she is adjusting to sleep deprivation and bleeding from a sore vagina and learning how to get milk from her breast to her baby. But because women do it every day, no one really talks about it at any length.

In that moment, though, I decide I don't know how to soothe my daughter.

"She hates me," I say aloud, so Chris will hear, so that everyone will hear, and Eula yanks off my nipple and stares up in my direction. She doesn't need to speak. I see in her eyes what she is saying. *C'mon, Mama, please do not take this all personally.* I am struck by my own immaturity again. Don't take any of it personally. Not this. Not my mom's comment about the luggage.

On this day of not taking anything personally, I walk Eula to the bathroom. I've got her in a football hold. She is wearing butterfly socks—black and white. We stand in front of the mirror.

"There you are, girl," I say.

She does not pay attention to her image; she looks up to the light fixture, notices only the light.

~

June calls me out of the cave.

It is time to birth myself back into the world. But it's a strange world to enter again. My shoulders have curled around my daughter. My eyes have become a telescope focused on one scene, my world small. Names of other places on the globe evaporate, country, continent, town. Is this how people become tribal and insular? My language has pared down.

I place Eula in her car seat and chug down the road. Just us. I am ready to feel autonomous as a woman in the woods with my daughter. Integrate back into the world. Come down from the astral plane. We are going to take ourselves up to a canyon to hike among lime-green leaves.

Everyone comments on her large cheeks.

They are my cheeks, straight from the DNA strand. When Pat-Pat saw a photo of me, her first grandchild, at eight months old, her words to my mother were:

"Oh gawd, look at those cheeks."

As if my cheeks were a problem. My mother still talks about it. "Can you imagine?" she says to me. "My first precious baby and *that* is what my mother says." I like to hear my mother defend me. I am already defending Eula's cheeks. I will take anyone down.

Eula agrees to face inward, to rest her gorgeous sweaty cheeks on my chest. I hold my breath with the ease of it. Please stay. Please stay. Sun pours through cottonwoods and dapples the ground. We pass an older couple hiking with poles, then a mountain biker. Dogs run past us. I am a woman walking in the woods with my sleeping baby. I am a woman walking in the woods with my sleeping baby. I am a woman walking in the woods with my sleeping baby. And I haven't peed. Is this actually happening? I could burst into a sprint. My feet could lift from the ground and take us to the golden dome of motherhood where, together, we will cartwheel and I will show Eula how to climb trees and roll down hills and jump rope and leap from just-high-enough places because I will be that mom who is body alive.

I start to make plans for everything we can do now.

As we approach the creek, I hear water rushing and stop. Do a Kegel. Do another Kegel, pulse them now. But it doesn't work. I let go. I let go right there. Pee runs down my legs. It soaks my pad. It overflows, breaks the dam through my pants and into my socks and into my shoes and down into the cracks of the ground. There is nothing I can do. Denial starts to creep toward me. I'm not a senior citizen. I cannot be incontinent. It must be temporary. Once we get past the newborn stage, my body will be fully healed. I rock my body back and forth and shush Eula and watch the coppery water of the creek flow by. I will walk the sticky mile back to my car. I wonder if any other new mothers walk around like this.

~

What I learn: The *wounded woman* archetype lives on the pocked streets of our every day. We are not immune from her. Should we be? I am not immune from her because I am her and—truth—have ached to become different iterations of her my entire life. We have grown up watching her in films, reading her in books, witnessing her in each other. Unlike other women, she is given cultural permission to lose control, go wild, and express the unexpressed. Of course, both men and women judge her for what appears to be weakness, but that doesn't stop her. Where does she come from? How old is she? When patriarchal rule swept over the world in the early 1200s, it began to overtake and bury land-based, matriarchal ways. This sounds like a gross overstatement. It's not. Mother Earth, and by proxy, women, became feared for their femaleness. Enter the dominator culture. Enter suppression. Enter extreme imbalance. Fast-forward to modern life where very little has changed. These days, in the coastal space of new motherhood, I stand on a weedy edge. What do I feel? What do I watch for? What has festered within me for years? Where am I in my conversation—because every woman is somewhere in her conversation—with the wounded woman?

~

Because we are a culture focused on the singular act of birthing, no one tells you what comes before or after birth. Not really. How can they? It's different for every woman. There may not be one narrative.

However, there is one truth. Before and after are not times where all you do is glow. These are passages full of rocks and caverns and shards of light. Maybe we protect the uninitiated women (and men). Maybe we hope they won't lose themselves like we did. Maybe time passes and we forget what we wanted to tell them in the first place.

Maybe we are scared to put the words *baby* and *hardship* in the same sentence.

During our final checkup, I lean toward my midwife and hide the subtle anxiety I am feeling with a joke.

"My vagina still feels like it's falling out. Seriously."

She assures me some new mothers feel this way. Somehow I grew into a body-focused thirty-three-year-old woman and didn't know this sort of thing happened at all, or was common. Do not worry. Oh, good. Even though I'm prone to pre-anticipate problems, I've assumed these physical issues fix themselves. I've had to in order to get through my days. I assume all the mothers out there are simply women who now walk around with a new demographic label: women-mothers. They may always have a belly pooch and wider hips, but I assume the body does eventually return. They run and leap and show their kids how to cartwheel. They make love. They walk twenty blocks no problem. They groove on the dance floor. They run marathons. They work manual labor. They scale mountains. They carry children and books and groceries and canoes and computers and bags of garden soil on their backs. They go back to moving like they used to.

I'm not wrong.

That is most often the case; or, it has been historically. But the path ahead for me will not be so textbook. My body has something else in mind. My body apparently needs to break down to get my attention.

I lie back for my internal exam. Chris dances around the room with Eula, swoops her up and down and sings to her. My midwife asks me to do a Kegel around her finger.

"Can you squeeze?" she says again.

"I did," I say, lifting my head. "I did, I am, can you feel it, I am right now, I can feel it, can you?"

"No, I can't. You have very little vaginal tone," she says.

"But *I* can feel my tone," I say. "Let me try again."

"It's okay, let's sit down."

We get comfortable on the couches. I reach my arms out for Eula and lead her to my breast. It's been six weeks. How could it be? I am ready to feel the collective warmth of leaving this pregnancy and birth journey on the high note of how easy and lucky breastfeeding has been for us, how healthy Eula is, how fine I am too. After a few wrap-up notes, our midwife shares how great it has been to work with us. Behind her smile, I can tell she has more to say; behind her calm voice is a seriousness I don't recognize yet. She writes down the name of a nurse who works for a urologist, a woman who is "really so nice."

I'm not sure why I need to see a specialist.

I don't know any other new mothers who have been to a specialist.

And why does she feel the need to tell me that she is really so nice?

I wait. I wait longer. Let the pause hover between us like a balloon.

The world before me goes blank. I can't locate myself in my own future.

She takes a breath.

"Molly, you have to trust that you *will* regain bladder control again, you *will* have satisfying orgasms again, you *will* feel strong again, you *will* experience vaginal tone again."

I nod my head.

I act as normal as you can act when a bus slams into you.

It hasn't occurred to me not to trust any of that until this exact moment when she tells me with such concrete sentences that I must trust it. Because now it's clear I've been in a sort of denial—a woman who has told herself all of the strange or bad would go away, away, away. Three days before Eula came into the world, I sat in the forest and made a verbal declaration about the birth: *I will soften and attune to my animal body and all will be well*. It's as if I called in what would be a continued request of myself from myself for years after.

I don't know where this all leads.

I'm not ready.

All will be well. But all is not well.

Little do I know this moment is the middle of the beginning of a two-year quest for my health, a crawl across the parched desert where I will question everything I once knew about my body, about what it means to heal, about the woman-mother I so wanted to become.

I'm about to lose my whole sense of self.

I'm about to pull those I love down with me.

I swallow, stand up, and thank her for her services with a hug.

When we walk out the door, I step into the sun a shattered woman.

The Girl Who Climbed Trees

On a brown porch, eucalyptus trees reached long scented leaves down to us two-year-olds. The dense forest called out—*Girls, girls, girls, be aware of what it means to be a girl.* We lived in Australia, on a continent made of songlines and the outlaws who paved over them. My friend started to cry and the prance in my legs slowed down. I didn't know why the tears but our adults moved around her like bees, humming, cooing, bending, and hugging. They tended to her unravel. Her blond curls everywhere. My brown curls limp.

This is my first memory.

This is where my body mythology began.

I had been born into a family of beautiful people. They considered me a beauty too—*those blue eyes, I love you in that smocked dress, you are so pretty, pretty girl.* We were internationals and yet we were traditional. My father went to work and provided. My mother stayed home with me (and then my brothers and me). She made dinner every night, stroked our foreheads with her smooth, cool hand, welcomed us with a bright smile, a new idea, how about we bang on pots to hear the sound? Her beauty was an important part of the familial equation. Corporate trips. Jewelry. So many silk scarves. Even when she got on her knees to scrub tiles, she never sweat or appeared disheveled. For my mother, self-decoration was an art, a pleasure of her own.

But my particular set of young eyes only saw the social agreement. Pretty Matters.

I wasn't one of those buttoned-up, tidy children. For my first five years, I knew only humid islands. When we lived in the Dominican Republic, near a busy dirt road where men sold avocados and hearts of palm, when we lived in a place where pale-skinned people like us had dark-skinned maids, a woman would come to our small stucco house to give my mother her weekly massage. The air clung to windows. It dripped down seams and pooled in cracks on the concrete patio. Curls matted to my forehead. Sticky was all I'd known. I stood in a doorway as my mother dropped her coral dress and draped her naked body over our wooden dining table. Like her own mother, she called her butt her "rear end." I plunked myself on the cool red tile floor underneath. Here I could be part of it all. My beautiful mother's red toenails on the edge.

I thought every mother must be a painting.

I thought every woman was meant to be a painting.

With my mother's family, beauty would become the ground cover of femaleness. My same-age cousin Lauren and I met on the steps of a cathedral in Chicago. Wind blew and papers skittered along the concrete. We could barely speak. With a bottle in one hand, she toddled toward me in pink satin. Someone nudged me forward in my white cotton. It was the start of her in dresses-that-poof and me in dresses-that-tie-in-the-back, her blond and my brown, her inhibition and my shy. She would become the closest thing I would ever have to a sister.

My body both wanted beauty and wanted to forget about beauty. Confused.

I grew into a girl with deer legs. We moved again. The willow tree outside our L-shaped house in Spain became my ally. Smells of laundry detergent wafted from our outdoor washing machine and my arms pulled me up branches. My legs latched. I hung upside down and inspected the dead crows below in our run-down pool. Hot breezes grazed against my brothers and me. From me, they learned to leap from limb to limb. Somewhere a family of iguanas trotted through the brittle grass. They didn't scare me. At our international school, the jungle gym was my home, climb higher, bend further, backflip off the swings.

My parents, though, might say I was a cautious child.

I was as reckless as a piece of toast.

I was as daring as a turtle.

But I was sure of how my body moved.

"Stop picking," my mom would say when my hands found knee scabs. I couldn't stop, though. What did these freckles on my body mean? What was that? Would my toe feel better after the bee sting and why did the bee sting make it hurt anyway? Was there a reason for that? I wanted to know all about my body. My mother interpreted my curiosity as worry. I interpreted her "Don't worry about it" as non-listening. It would take years to develop the language to correct each other.

I made plans for the strong woman I would become.

Fast runner.

Tree leaper.

My sneakers crunched on the gravel of our schoolyard. My friends and I sized each other up without knowing we were doing so. I wanted to rub my body against my blond friend—to get as close as possible to her face, mouth, hair, to play house and cave with her, as if our closeness would make me more like her. My arms clung around her neck at birthday parties. I would not release her. I wanted to make her mine, make me her, make her me.

Meanwhile, my mother lifted heavy things. She hauled terra-cotta pots. I saw her kill spiders, lug bags and bags of groceries, and muscle large bottles of drinking water from car to house. Once, when we drove up to a dead horse on a dirt road, she got out to inspect, swatted flies, and told us horrified kids it was fine. She rarely asked for help from a man. She never shrieked. Somehow she did it all while wearing a pear-shaped ivory necklace and pants that never smeared with dirt. When my parents hosted dinner parties, Fleetwood Mac played loud on my father's stereo and she appeared from behind our bamboo furniture like a doll.

Lipstick.

Clothes ironed.

Big white smile on her pretty moon face.

On one of our summer vacations to Illinois, my parents gave me a Get-in-Shape Girl kit for my seventh birthday. The 1980s had provided it, everything I had ever wanted in a gift. Lauren and I darted around on soft grass all day. Smells of boat gasoline and lake water and sunscreen stuck to our girl skin—then Lauren got sick and went to the doctor and I was left to play with the set of small weights, jump rope, wristbands, and cassette tape. Under the oak trees, I pumped iron in the proper amount of reps. Be as strong as a gymnast. In America, on magazine covers at the grocery store, blond women posed with blank looks on their faces. In my cultural home context that was the definition of beauty. I wanted strength instead, but also whatever it was that would make me desirable. Later, when Lauren came back, we flopped belly-down on the grass in our green and pink swimsuits, our legs stretched long behind us, our faces pressed together. In her husky woman voice, Lauren told me she wanted to be just like someone called Marilyn Monroe and that she had been practicing how to French kiss with her pillow. I pretended to know what she was talking about.

Back overseas, I greeted my backyard full of lizards and porcupines, led my animal figurines outside for fresh air, and got back on my bike. We were surrounded by low hills. The sun warmed my legs as I tested my speed. Freedom spread over me again and my eyes closed to take it all in. Then my face hit gravel. I stood up, tasted blood in my mouth, and ran with my hands out toward the house, screaming. At the hospital, I lay on a gurney in the hallway and stared at aqua-colored tiled walls. My parents whispered nearby. Eventually, the doctor stood over me and announced they wouldn't have to stitch it.

The skin flap that attached my top lip to gum would grow back.

"Let's go home," I said. My brothers had cracked their heads open on pool edges and rocks. They knew about stitches. Not me. After sundown, tucked into my yellow bed, I touched my mouth and absorbed a new electric knowledge.

The body could heal on its very own.

This was how the body worked.

My mood, unlike my brothers' moods, shifted based on how my body felt. That would become truer and truer as I grew up. These were the surest years of my life—two to three to four to five to six to seven to eight years old. My name was Molly May and I was an older sister and I had brown hair and blue eyes and I wanted to live in trees. Only from a great long distance was I aware of what it meant to be in a human body that was specifically girl.

Amass

The nurse at the urology office *is* nice, super nice. Now that I understand the incontinence might be real, I'm trying to be an adult and gather data. In the tiny examination room, she chit-chatters and snakes a painful catheter up my urethra. My body retracts, suddenly remembers I had one at the end of Eula's birth.

"Ow," I say. "Ow, ow, ow, ow."

It's the only way I know how to say *Please stop* without being rude.

"Oh, I'm so sorry," she says, and she pulls it out. "We can use a thinner one."

After we sort out the catheter, she puts electrodes on my low hips, vagina, and anus and then hooks me up to a machine. She explains how to do a proper Kegel—imagine you are sucking a straw up your butt. This is useful information. I can do that. In my blue paper gown, I practice, and we watch the monitor together. The lines peak up and go down. We might be watching for an earthquake.

"Good job," she says. "See, you've got some tone there." She becomes my cheerleader but, since pregnancy, I don't have much drive. I'm tired. I glance at my watch.

"Thank you for showing me this," I laugh. "Now I *really* understand Kegels."

We laugh together.

"Oh, I need to be home in half an hour to nurse my daughter," I say as if I've just realized it, as if the thought of it isn't the foreground to every minute of my day.

Once I'm dressed, we go over our findings. We've established that I have a low-grade cystocele (prolapse of the bladder) and rectocele (prolapse of the rectum). The word *prolapse* is familiar to me. One of my best friends has one from her first child's birth. My mother has one. When I was in college, she told me about her upcoming surgery to fix the issue of a "bulge" protruding out of her vagina. I pretended not to be scared by this older-woman problem. She was never incontinent from it, though. A few years later, her rectocele relapsed. That's the last I'd heard about it.

But what is the bulge? What is falling out of what? When the pelvic floor loses strength and suppleness, it can no longer hold the organs (uterus, bladder, rectum, and small bowel) in place. So one or many can get misaligned and fall into and *bulge* against the vaginal canal or anus. This creates pressure and discomfort. Sometimes an organ actually droops out of one of those openings. I'm not at that point. Thank goodness.

I learn the word *prolapse* means "to fall out of place."

I try not to double down on the meaning.

"You know," says the nurse, "we can try to fit you for a pessary. It will change your world."

"What is it?"

"It's like a diaphragm," she says and pulls out a pamphlet to show me how it holds the cystocele in place so large amounts of urine don't pour out of you due to impact, walking, any strenuous activity.

"I'm open to it." I hesitate. "But I'm such a low-maintenance person, I don't like extra things, or devices. I don't know if it makes sense for me, and is it possible that it could prevent actual healing?"

"I think we should try it. You love to hike. You've said that's really important to you. What can happen is a woman stops doing the things she loves because she is worried about peeing. And if she stops doing the things she loves, then she is missing a big part of who she is and that can lead to other issues. So let's get you out hiking, and wearing your daughter, like you want to."

"Okay," I say, and smile.

I rush back home. When Eula latches to my breast, I wonder how it's possible to be treated so kindly by someone and yet feel invaded, actually assaulted, by the process.

On our next visit, the nurse and I spend two hours together.

She helps me squat and put the latex cup inside my vagina. I've warmed to the idea of it. It *could* change my world. We jump up. I haven't jumped since giving birth. I am sure I will split in half. But I don't. One size is too big, the other too small, and by the end, my vagina feels sore, raw, done, done with this trying on. The nice nurse bends the office rules and lets me take both pessaries home. Try them out. Go on walks. Go wild, she tells me. Leap around. Bring the one that doesn't work back. When she leans over paperwork to help me figure out how to make sure insurance pays for all these visits, I want to collapse in her kind lap.

Instead I utter *Thank you, thank you, thank you* until she tells me to stop.

"You're such a beautiful young mother," she says. "You shouldn't have to deal with any of this."

Is that what I am?

I don't know what I am these days.

And, really, no one should have to deal with any of this.

"Let me know how it goes," she says, and hands me the paper bag.

~

What I learn: Most women don't know about the pelvic bowl. How is this possible? We use it all the time and have no idea we are using it. It is not part of our American education. We do not learn it in anatomy or sex ed classes. Gynecologists don't talk about it unless something has gone wrong. Even birth classes only seem to mention it in passing: "Do a Kegel from time to time." Our mothers don't share it with us because no one shared it with them. No one *knows*. Or, no one *speaks* of it. I started to read about the pelvic bowl in my early thirties only because a friend gave me a book. It was a theory to me. I did a few visualizations. That was it. Pelvic-floor disorders are a huge unspoken global health problem for hundreds of millions of women around the world. In low-resource countries, women who experience prolonged obstructed labor end up with a fistula or hole between vagina and another organ, leading to fecal and/or urinary incontinence. Then, because of how they smell, these women are usually ostracized from their communities, seen as dirty, no longer accepted, no options at all.

So, women birth the next generation (if the baby lives) and then get ousted.

How is this okay?

Women's pelvic health isn't even a concept in most countries. In France, and other parts of Europe, though, women can go to postnatal vaginal toning class paid for by Social Security. I see a direct correlation between awareness and support for the pelvis and cultural body shame. Americans are behind. We recognize there is a problem, but our government sure isn't going to pay for it. Private health insurance doesn't either.

My American midwife was revolutionary for sending me to a specialist.

We should all be sent to specialists.

It should be a normalized regime during postpartum regardless of any birth complications.

Female anatomy, considered a nether region, has always been less studied. *Pudenda* means the external genital organs, especially those of the female. This Latin word means "shame." Language reflects what we value and what we don't. There is a mass disconnect from a part of us so essential to well-being. Our power source is on lockdown—a secret underused. What if, early on, girls learned about the pelvic bowl as a place to care for, a place to ask questions of?

I'm interested in body fluency.

Imagine if the world was made up of people fluent in their own bodies.

~

Now that Eula is no longer technically a newborn, are we no longer newborn into parenthood? I watch Chris swaddle her, tuck the muslin tight around her body, and coo into her ear. He seems generally unfazed. Lack of sleep puffs his eyes. But at night, he rises like a soldier on duty to change her diaper and place her back in the nook of my arm. He also isn't lactating or going through a major hormonal change or healing process or recovery from pregnancy. But I can't see that context yet. His ability to work with his hands translates into his new role as Papa.

He broke ground on our house the other day.

He plans to build it on his own, with occasional help from his brother or the hiring of a carpenter friend. It's a small house but a huge project. Though we've never operated with prescribed gender roles, we are now—woman cares for babe, man builds shelter. I recognize the pressure on him. He needs to be all of it. It's a new masculine for our generation: listener, worker, active parent, part provider, sensitive, but strong still, whatever *strong* means. Next to our bed, there are stacks of books from the library: plumbing, slab floors, how to wire your house. He reads them by headlamp before bed, this man who teaches himself everything. I try to tell him as often as possible that he's amazing. My mother calls him the absentminded professor. He's a problem solver who can fix almost anything but sometimes forgets to turn off the stove, close the refrigerator, or put the top back on an ink pen.

Our first sex since birth was slow and exploratory. It broke a new sort of seal, but wasn't painful at all. We both wondered whether orgasm would happen for me ever again. It wasn't my usual swift river current. It didn't narrow and widen. It didn't leap over an edge. Instead, it was everywhere—an ocean of small waves, then a settle down and then more small waves and then settle and more small waves.

"Strange, almost too much to feel," I whispered.

"Just feel into it," he encouraged.

It gave me some hope.

One morning, I explain to Chris that neither pessary works.

"Well," he says, "I think you have to treat healing your pelvic floor like it's physical therapy."

"Yeah, except it's my vagina, my bladder. It's demoralizing."

"But it's like any other part of the body, Molly," he says. "You have to do exercises and then it'll get better."

I can't be so practical right now.

I stomp away to the corner of our living space with Eula in my arms. He continues making his oatmeal. As usual, he retreats and avoids battle. I stare out the window and, within minutes, come upon the best analogy. I've got it. Won't threaten him. He'll understand this way.

"So," I say with a neutral voice, turning back toward him, "I have a great way to explain it. Imagine you've been working hard to build a house for us, just like my body grew and brought Eula into the world for us. Well, what if you fell off the ladder and broke your leg, except somehow it's a body part as intimate as your penis . . . and it got so bad there was a threat of amputation and you had this potentially permanent wound from your efforts to do something for our family. That would be hard. That's how I feel right now."

"*Molly*," he says, almost laughs.

"What?"

"That doesn't work. You can't use that. There are many factors you aren't considering in our conflict."

My body snaps to attention, starts to plate itself with heavy armor. I'm supposed to take a deep breath in a moment like this but I forget what I'm supposed to do. We have been in a transition. Over a year ago, he told me there had never been a safe space in our marriage for him to have an opposite opinion or a voice. I listened, felt bad about myself, and then jumped into action. We had the noble and impossible intention of sorting out these issues before parenthood—meaning, during what would be my easy pregnancy. Despite a pregnancy that felt like an illness, I found bursts of energy for therapy and setting intentions. Meanwhile, part of me scratched at my insides, wanted to scream, and then did scream, "But what about me?" Got desperate. Wanted the occasional foot rub. Wanted attention. Wanted to be seen and soothed. Wanted him to stop drinking his beloved coffee because the smell of it made me vomit instantly and, when he did stop, I swore the smell was still lodged in his pores, demanded he take a shower before he came close to me. I craved closeness. I created isolation upon isolation. It's hard, he told me, to move toward a person who snarls.

"I know. But this is a specific moment in time," I say now, my shoulders braced. "Can't you just hear me out on that example?"

"It is impossible for me to be compassionate when you are angry. This is an old pattern of ours and . . ." he says with a voice so sterile it might hurt me more than what he is actually saying, "I can't give into it anymore."

I set Eula down on the bed and pull sandals onto my feet.

I don't know where I'm going but I'm leaving.

I don't know how to leave with a baby in my arms.

"It would help me, one day, in some far distant future," I say, and let him hear my choke, ". . . if you were capable of saying, *I'm sorry this is so hard. Thank you for bringing our daughter into the world. It must be so hard to feel your body suffering.*"

He doesn't have time to answer because I'm out the door with Eula.

We nestle down by the creek. Maybe the rushing water will cure me of everything. We are less than fifty feet from the guesthouse. I don't want my parents to see me. I don't want him to find us. He won't come looking anyway. Eula stares up at the flick of cottonwoods. There is so much green.

"Sometimes parents argue, sweets," I say to her. "It's okay."

She just watches me, watches the world.

For over a decade, he has said yes to me.

Now he is saying no.

I understand the need for this change.

But the timing is awful. Didn't we deal with all that drama during my pregnancy? Wasn't I done with being the angry woman? Wasn't he going to engage me more, be a better listener? The creek wants me to remember simplicity. It knows I know it has the answer. Rocks and stones gaze up at me like a group of wet people. Cold water numbs my feet, blurry over my sandals. I want to pout, even though everything about this creek moment reminds me about the great circle, the ebb, the flow, the let go, that everything does and will wash away and become something new. Don't give me your truth right now, nature. I want to dwell on the fact that I'm starting to see men as less than.

I cannot distinguish between what irritation is appropriate for me to feel and not.

I am a walking contradiction.

The next day we get together with women from our birth class—
The Milk Bar. We nurse our babes on couches and share. I want to be
honest. I'm not interested in pretend or saving face. Ha, ha, I laugh
about my incontinence because that's all I can do. No one else is peeing on herself. Are we all in a private vortex? I take Eula's tiny pants
off to change her diaper and say, aloud, "Let's show off these thighs."

What kind of mother says that? Sometimes I don't know why
what comes out of my mouth comes out of my mouth. I am always the
strange one. I was never going to be a mother who cared about being
like other mothers.

My black-haired babe stares up at me.

We are here together, she tells me.

You and me. Do not worry.

I don't know who thought it was a good idea to put me in charge
here.

~

During the last incontinence visit my health insurance allows, the
nice nurse seems puzzled the pessary didn't work. I hope it's all a
mistake, wrong fit, but no. She confirms it must have to do with the
structure of my anatomy. My body is one of those bodies that just
wouldn't accept it.

"There are other options," she says.

"I'm not into intervention."

"I know you aren't, but I want you to know about all of them. You
have to be done having children to have surgery . . ."

The word *surgery* catapults me to the moon. It is cold up here, a
calm blackness, black upon black upon black sky, and, far away, small
spots shimmer.

When I descend, she is explaining something about a sling or net.

"Is this common?" I interrupt her.

"What?"

"Incontinence for mothers my age."

"Most of my patients are older women, but, remember, you had
a vacuum delivery. That can change things. Some young moms leak

when they sneeze, but you have a few extra challenges. You need to take your Kegels seriously."

"Here," she says, and hands me a huge catalogue for incontinence pads with images of elderly women wearing khakis and smiling in landscaped parks. "These pads are thicker. They'll be better than any pad you can buy at the drug store."

I nod.

Maybe distraction is the best tactic here, but I'm not made that way.

Some of us coast. Some of us excavate. Some of us do both. I had been a shiny metal excavator my entire life: unearthed every small seed and gnarled root and then assigned meaning to them. I will not take anything, especially a diagnosis, at face value. I have to believe my body can heal without a quick fix. There *has* to be a way to retrain my pelvic bowl, my ligaments, my whatever. There is some lesson for me here. I will develop endurance for it. I can do endurance.

Must operate this way.

I cannot be a young woman who wears pads made for an old woman.

I cannot turn toward that reality.

"Also," she says with panda bear eyes, "something told me to give you this poem. It might help. It made me think of you. It's called 'She Let Go.'"

She puts the photocopy into my hand.

I give her a hug and thank her.

It takes effort to ignore the start of my plummet downward.

Outside the brick hospital building, magpies hop and squawk on a nearby sidewalk. They call and respond to the bright day. I pause, tuck the poem into my back pocket, and toss the pad catalog into a trash can.

~

My mom and I decide to take Eula to the farmer's market. It will be one of my first outings to a public place at about two months postpartum. On the long drive across the valley, my child turns into a werewolf. She wails and her little mouth won't stop. I lean over her in the backseat.

"It's okay, sweet love," I whisper, but all I'm really thinking is *I don't know if I can love you if you are like this all the time.* It occurs to me she might be screaming because her mother can't fully relax these days. I want to discard some rhetoric in one camp of parenting, the one I tend to follow. It says Eula is imprinting on my every momentary emotion.

Let's go ahead and blame the mother. Tell the pregnant woman she must eat, feel, and birth perfectly for the well-being of the fetus. She inevitably fails at this but still holds out hope she will be a glowing mother of her baby. Then, at the peak of her sleep deprivation, possible vaginal collapse, physical depletion from nursing, and isolation from a partner who doesn't "get it," she gets a little angry at the world. But do not feel your anger, honey. Transmute it with breathing exercises and yoga you can't do because you either can't move that way anymore or there is no extra time. Become superhuman, even though no one is meant to be not human. Whatever you do, do not expose your dear baby to your darkness. You are not allowed to have darkness.

Bullshit.

Sounds like a military operation.

I want my daughter to know we all feel a range of emotions.

But I do believe she's imprinting on me. I do.

The farmer's market is packed and loud. So much kale, lettuce, so many bunches of radishes, so many people. People skip along, tasting, laughing, cash in hand. I stroll and hope I don't see anyone I know. Eula nuzzles into my wrap but I'm not sure how long she'll be quiet and content without me bouncing. My mother darts in and out of stands, filling her canvas bag with vegetables. She is an expert at efficiency. She is food as healing. She practices Ayurveda. Around her, I become more a girl, less a woman and less capable. Is it because she is so capable? This is the gold, a friend told me, to be living with my mother while becoming a mother. I know it's true. I know this is how humans have lived for millennia. But I don't want to lean on her too much.

Maybe it's okay to be less capable.

She wants to get Korean food.

The line is long.

I tell her if Eula starts to cry I will walk back to the car and wait there.

I tell her if pee breaches my pad I will walk back to the car and wait there.

"Are people looking at me?" I ask her.

"No, why?" she asks.

"I don't know. Are my pants see-through, did I already pee on them?" I whisper. "I feel like everyone is staring at me."

"No, Moll," she says. "You are just a beautiful woman walking with her newborn." Some days I want to marry my mother.

~

At home, I borrow my mother's Caroline Myss books. Mine are asleep in a cardboard box with my other books in storage. We have shared her work for years. My mother relates because Myss, like her, is a Catholic from Chicago. As a self-described medical intuitive and mystic, Myss is no-nonsense, direct, a kind bully.

"Your biography becomes your biology," she writes.

I don't need to be coerced into believing so.

It's tricky, though. It's almost offensive. It could border on self-blame. It puts illness right back into the person's hands, encourages a deeper look. Chris always speaks up on this conversation; he says sometimes people get sick just because they get sick, it doesn't have to be some trauma from childhood or some unreleased emotion. He recognizes the wormhole for people like me.

I agree and don't agree with him.

I believe in agency.

In the early night hours of Eula's sleep, I read and scribble notes in my journal. We have begun a slow dance—my health data and me. Sometimes I want to clutch it close and accept its flaws so we can move beyond with grace together. Other times, its stank breath makes me lean far back and avoid eye contact. But we can't leave each other and so the push and pull unfolds. It is time, again, to become a geographer of my body. Isn't it what I've always wanted?

Become both the traveler and the map.

Become both the traveler and the map.

It is the only way.

~

The early summer rain streaks the sky purple. Eula and I sit under a cottonwood tree by the creek. Leaves rustle. She smiles at me a thousand times, burrows into my chest, and falls asleep for two hours.

It's never happened before—this easy sleep.

I want to be nothing but her mother. She has learned to fall asleep without motion. My energy rises. Everything will change for the better now. I don't yet know that babies are like adults, full of moods and impermanent actions.

I'm so glad I eat two bars of chocolate.

Later that afternoon, Eula spits my nipple out. Over the bathroom sink, I hand-express it out, watch white heads of milk form on my nipple and drip down and away. Go away, chocolate. It takes trial and error to figure out what food passes through me and upsets her stomach.

At night, we draw our wool curtains, turn on ocean sounds, and put Eula to sleep in her co-sleeper next to our bed. Because the guesthouse is one room, we are held hostage by this rhythm. If we click on a stove to cook, she wakes up. If my toes crack, she rouses. Somehow she tolerates the sound of our quiet voices. We exist in whispered dark from eight o'clock onward.

My mother brings roast chicken and salad over to us for dinner.

Again.

My incontinence, though I haven't fully shared the degree of it with my parents, has ratcheted me into a sort of invalid. I'm unable to do anything but care for Eula. Not cook. Not clean. Not even put a respectable outfit on my body. I eat crackers all day long. Some might call this a depression, but I don't go there. During one of Eula's short naps, I ate bread so quickly and spilled an entire bowl of olive oil on my computer and now one-third of the letters don't work.

I have no idea what Chris eats.

"Here you go," my mother says to us as we huddle together in the kitchen.

"Thank you so much," I whisper, and continue to pace around, telling them both I need to tend to my eating habits, maybe this is step one of healing.

"Cooking has never been your favorite thing," Chris says.

"That isn't true. I spent a whole summer growing, harvesting, blanching, and freezing Swiss chard and kale."

"I know," he says, and plays it safe by saying nothing else. Everyone in this room knows food can be a complication for me. I grew and cared for all those vegetables but never ate any of them.

"Maybe I can help you stock your pantry," my mom offers.

This is her domain. My cells are made of her green soup, her spicy rice dishes, her love put on the table for all of us. As a young woman, I made a choice to be less domestic and more intellectual: toast and salad all day long so my mind could explore. It never occurred to me that they could coexist. I don't want to pass my food issues on to my daughter. Colorful food actually brings me deep satisfaction and joy. I have to change now. My mother rocks in the rattan bamboo chair and listens to me say nothing.

What is motherhood even?

I don't want my mother's exact version.

I want my own.

I stay awake that night. Flat on my back in bed, I watch the trees beyond our window reach up to a dark sky—one hand on my daughter to check her breath, another hand on my man to feel his chest rise and fall, my ears listen for my dog snoring beneath our bed. Then a great wave washes over me and we float on the sea and move together, and all because I am an octopus with a limb on everyone, my eyes wide now to the ceiling, to be sure of everyone, because someone has to be, because someone wants to be, and that someone now is me.

~

Sleep becomes a state of the past.

Chris reminds me that lack of sleep affects mood. I don't have the presence of mind to connect that sleep deprivation also affects my ability to muster the gusto to heal myself.

I cannot sleep because I cannot stop listening to my daughter.

On the days Eula falls asleep under trees on my chest, I am a complete mother. But to walk with her on me for every nap hurts my pelvic floor. Usually I have to swaddle and sing and bounce her for an indoor nap. When she eventually goes down, I collapse in a chair to decide what to do with my time: change my pad, eat an entire container of dates, write emails, read a book from the stack, pick my new toe wart, stare at the wall, or do my Kegels. My Kegels come and go. They aren't hard exercises. But I may as well be hauling my heart up a frozen mountain.

She never sleeps long. Half an hour max. On the rare day, she dozes for two hours and, despite my laments about no self-time, I spend those extra minutes sitting next to her, watching her sleep, willing her to wake up because I miss her.

~

What I learn: In pregnancy, you spend almost ten months opening your belly and pelvis. Afterward, they still feel open. Come back in; contract back in. For thousands of years, indigenous people have had traditions for helping a new mother seal her body back together and tone stretched abdominal muscles—*sarashi* in Japan, *fajas* in Latin American cultures, *rebozos* in Mexico, and the Malaysian Bengkung are some. Long strips of cloth are wound tightly around a woman's midsection after birth. This is not cosmetic. This practice knits muscles back together (can heal a diastasis recti) and helps a woman feel emotionally contained again.

I am not indigenous to anywhere I can name. Neither are most of my people. My people have no taproot tradition around pregnancy, birth, or motherhood other than passing on tips about sleep and work-life balance. My people live in small houses with small nuclear families, almost never in a shared-housing situation. My people cannot walk down the road to the comfort of an old friend's porch because my people don't live where they grew up. My people usually don't have time for a spontaneous conversation because there isn't much spaciousness in life. They can't linger much. They are scheduled down to the hour by work, family, and self-improvement, even when they freelance life. My people want to be good. They don't want to get trapped or weighted down even though they sometimes are. My people are obsessed with finding *balance*, the very thing once embedded and foundational and therefore once not in need of a name. My people are aware of the rhythm they live by. They feel it's necessary. They don't want to be limited by old ways, though they recognize a loss. Maybe we respond to the needs of our era. Maybe we are all some form of the ouroboros—a snake on the grand chase for its own tail.

~

Almost every week, we have walked in the woods with Holcomb. Sometimes we meet at a gas station, put the babes in one car, and hope they don't cry on the way to the trailhead—her daughter bleats like a lamb; mine wails like a banshee. When we hop out, the scent of living plants knocks me over backward, right into the skin of my old self. We enter the forest and bow. The forest bows back. It will all be okay. I know myself here among trees. But am I on the ground yet, after these months? Some part of me hovers, tethered still to that astral plane of labor and birth. Green cottonwoods and dark firs lean in and flutter, *Hello.*

"I *love* nature," I say with no other vocabulary for what I mean.

"It's essential," she says back.

We walk and discuss.

What would it be like to keep on walking and never return to this mothering life?

What would it be like to be a father instead of a mother?

What would happen if our husbands could spend just one day in our bodies?

What would we give for a week of full nights of sleep? Really. Make a list.

What is going on?

What is going on?

Where is the tribe?

Why do people live so far away from each other?

How are we capable of so much love, it hurts almost, doesn't it?

How many ounces come out when you pump? Does it even work?

Isn't it brutal that we can't eat the chocolate that soothes us because it upsets our daughters?

Do your dreams alarm you?

I make a conscious decision to ask Holcomb almost no questions about my body issues right now. She is my doctor and she's on maternity leave. I don't want to saturate our friendship or her postpartum time with work talk. She senses though and asks me questions. I give her the gist, downplay, and redirect. A few years ago, pre-babes, when she did her first women's exam on me, she asked me to squeeze around her finger.

"Whoa," she had said, "that might be the strongest vaginal tone I've ever felt."

The irony.

We sit on twisted logs in shade to nurse our babes. Holcomb's nipples are shredded from her daughter's lip-tie; every single latch sends searing pain through her breast. But she is determined to continue and will. Most mamas would have stopped. I probably would have stopped. We wonder at our own woman-ness. She tells me she sneezed once and leaked and can't believe that is a constant experience for me. We woman each other up as best we can.

We strap our daughters back into the front carriers.

Eula won't face my chest and be legal according to the safety rules of carriers. My rebel child. I accommodate and flip her around so her eyes can steer out to the world. Face out. I hold the neck she can't fully hold up yet and watch my feet as we continue.

Don't fall.

Don't fall over a root.

By the end of each walk, my legs are sticky with urine, despite my tactic to drink almost no water. The downhill makes it hard to avoid. It becomes a situation I start to accept and prepare for with a plastic sheet already placed on the driver's seat. When we say goodbye to Holcomb in the hot dusty trailhead parking lot, I laugh about my wet pants, a mere annoyance.

I cannot let the shock in.

It would swamp me out of being able to drive my car straight on the road, arrive home, take my daughter out of her car seat, unpeel my clothes, rinse off in the shower, put her down for a nap with patience, do dishes, prepare for returning to writing work with clients, and try to be a decent partner to the man who made her with me.

~

But sometimes, at night, fear flaps awake in my chest again. Don't be in denial. Don't. I email my midwife to ask for a reference to a pelvic therapist, someone who can give me a range of concrete exercises and see me through to an end. I need to amass more information and prepare for some kind of future with it.

At the pelvic therapist's office, I sit in my car and tell myself this is it. Get serious now. It's like healing any other body part. Freedom will be delivered to me in a package of three to five exercises. I walk into the gym-type physical therapy place for the first time. Other people are here to tend to torn hamstrings and sprained ankles. Not vaginas. Maybe that normalizes it.

She is so perky. I get intimidated by blond perky people. Be open. Act open.

"Let's go to the back room," she says, and I follow her, stare at her tan legs, and start to make up all the reasons her life must be easy. By the time we get to The Back Room, I've coached myself down from acting like an insecure seventh grader.

She gives me a tampon-sized sensor and I joke that I don't need to walk down the hallway to the bathroom to insert it. I'll just do it here. I'm past the point of privacy. But when she breaks eye contact, I realize I'm breaking a rule and she's uncomfortable.

When I return from the bathroom, the little monitor clues me in to how strong my pelvic-floor contractions are.

"Good job," she says to me, as I lie on the massage table and watch green lines go up and down, another personal seismograph.

I start to like her. She's here to help after all. I want to believe that someone who has never given birth or had pelvic-floor issues can help me with my pelvic floor. In theory, this should be easy to believe.

I come back once a week. My contractions improve slightly. But when they don't improve for a few weeks and she seems aloof and sort of not in it anymore, I explain that I'm overwhelmed and sometimes I get angry about the whole thing and sabotage myself and don't do my exercises at home, especially when I haven't slept more than two hours at night. We are past her realm of expertise, but it doesn't stop me from sharing. She can see the wild in my eyes, and I can see in her eyes that she has never experienced the wild for herself.

I know it's not nice but I decide she's too vanilla for me and I'm too volcanic for her. It's the easiest feeling to feel in that moment. Chris will plant a gentle question: do you think you are sabotaging yourself even more by not going back? Nope. No more visits to the The Back Room for me.

~

Because I can no longer control my urine, I try to control the person who loves me the most. My mother tells me I'm a great mother one day. The next day, I rip her apart for her mothering of me. The smallest infractions create a tornado within me. I don't know who I am.

"Eula sure does frown a lot," she says as we stand in her kitchen.

"It's not a frown, Mom, it's a furrow of the brow," I explain.

"Oh please, Molly."

"Language matters," I snap back. "I know you don't think about language, but it *does* matter. Eula isn't expressing distaste or upset with that look. It's her look of curiosity. Chris does the same thing with his brow. It would be helpful if her family would actually take note of what she is trying to communicate."

There is a deeper layer about me feeling unseen and unwitnessed when I tried to communicate as a girl. We don't talk about that.

"Okay, whatever," she says, and she sighs. "I'm sorry."

My mother comes from the land of Deal-With-It. She spent her early motherhood schlepping three children (alone, usually) around the world, boiling drinking water, and negotiating for medicine in second-world countries without getting to process her feelings. I come from the privileged land of Question-It. Please put me in the murky water so I can know it and taste it and become more textured for it and push an edge so others can push the edge one day too. I don't know where our territories overlap.

I also know how to deal.

I take Eula for the first time to one of my doctor's visits. The flowing waterfall in the waiting room keeps her attention for our long wait. It's my toe, some strange cyst/blister/wart thing that apparently comes with pregnancy. The dermatologist asks me how we want to do this.

"Just give me a sec," I tell her, and I sit upright, in a half ab-crunch, to latch Eula onto my breast. I am proud for being so calm, for wearing a pad and not worrying about pee. When the needle goes into my foot, I gasp and squeeze her diapered bum and she smiles up at me.

The cauterizing takes longer.

The room smells of burnt skin.

"Do you smell your mama's skin burning?" I ask Eula.

Later that night, we put Eula down, hook up the monitor, and walk from the dark guesthouse to a cabin full of light for dinner. I tell my family I want to wean Eula from the pacifier during her nap. My mother tells me not to *fret*.

"I'm not fretting," I say.

"Yes, you are," she says.

"No," I counter, as my father and Chris scuttle to the other side of the room, "I'm paying attention to my child. I'm watching her spit her pacifier out routinely and making the assumption this means she might be done, so let me seize that moment. I'm actually super aware of her responses and setting intentions for how to move forward. And if you think I'm trying to control something, yes, I am. I'm trying to control some part of my chaotic life right now. I'm trying to prevent further disaster. I'm trying my best."

I know I sound mean. I don't care.

No one continues the conversation. It doesn't elude me that I can express my rage here only because my family culture has created a safe space. My mother, if she had anger, never had that space herself. So few women do. My people have not shut my vocalization down. I can speak my truth to Chris because I know he won't beat me or leave me if I do. This creates a watery moat of allowance around me. But that doesn't make it fair for them. I know it's not bad to feel what I feel. I will stand up for the importance of actually feeling it and expressing. But I recognize that my irritation is mostly misdirected; this compounds my remorse; this release in the wrong direction is hard for me to change in the moment, even when I try, because it begs to land somewhere and I don't know where else it can land.

Loved ones surround me but I feel like an island, unsupported.

They are all against me.

They are all against me.

When I slink back to bed that evening, sobs move through my body. Chris spoons me. When he cannot settle me, he starts to climb onto me, to get close, as close as possible, as if his wife is a bull who has lost her compass. My mouth takes the shape Eula's does when she cries. Because I feel tenderness for her in those moments, I am tender, for a moment, toward myself. It's a strange new relationship.

~

My friends ask whether it was love at first sight. When the nurses took Eula from me, I followed her with my eyes but didn't *know* this creature who had just slipped from my womb. I loved her in the way a young wolf loves her pups—heart kicks into instinct and she protects and nurtures without having known how to do so beforehand. It took us a few days to master our latch. I was her food. I wanted to be her food. We grew into a rhythm with each other, with her arm flung over my breast, her eyes closed, sometimes open and watching me. Any time I tried to remove her for any reason, she would ninja block me with her tiny hand.

Now we are old pros.

Eula makes a certain whimper, paws at me, and I lift or unbutton my shirt. She is still part of my body. We are of one body. My mother breastfed me for six weeks and then had to stop. I was losing weight. She couldn't get the proper latch and no one showed her how to latch. The nurses also told her some women aren't *successful* at it and didn't encourage her to continue. I don't think I knew this until recently. But it comes up often these days. She is reliving her early motherhood as she watches me live mine.

One of my mother's close friends comes over.

We sit under cottonwoods for a splotch of shade on this bright summer day. These older women gurgle at Eula as she nurses.

"Look at her," they both murmur.

"I know," I say, and smile back.

I start to tell them about what I've recently learned about mother's milk because it's new to me. I never read books about it while pregnant and had rarely been around mothers and new babies.

"Mother's milk is about way more than food. It's about connection and safety and bonding. It's obvious but isn't that amazing?"

"Yeah," my mother says, with sunscreen smeared and sweating in white lines down her face.

"Well," she adds, "when we moved across the world, my milk dried up."

It was the stress. She moved from Australia to the Dominican Republic when my younger brother was barely a month old. He went on formula too. She wishes someone had been around to encourage her to keep trying with my brother, with me.

Two opposing thoughts emerge for me.

She is a badass, far stronger than I will ever be.

She could have made an effort to find someone to help her.

"I feel grateful that it's been so easy for us," I say.

"Breastfeeding sets the tone for the relationship," my mother's friend adds. Maybe she is saying that to make me feel good, but I don't like it. I think of all my friends who haven't been able to nurse, and what I become is a woman with a sword ready to defend my mother.

I am starting to understand that what women say they do as mothers is a thing.

In that silent space between sentences, a bird lifts off a branch, a creek stone dislodges and rushes downstream, a coyote somewhere stalks across a field, and I can feel my mother feeling me and me feeling her and then almost at the same time, in one swell, we all say the same exact phrase, the only true phrase out there.

"But mothers do the best they can with what they have."

~

In my mother's bathroom, I find her Mason Pearson hairbrush. It is sleek and black. I've just taken a bath and she lounges in the living room with Eula. She has always told me that it's the best brush—no hair snag, gentle, made from some amazing material. Yeah, whatever, Mom, I've thought. I don't need a fancy hairbrush. I don't need to pay that much for my hair. But now, standing naked on the wood floor, I want this brush. I want all of my mother's beauty tips. Not because I fear I am aging but because she is aging. And I haven't listened to anything. I haven't listened to anything. Oh god, I haven't listened to anything about anything from her.

~

"Remember when we went to church?" I say.

"Yeah," my mother responds, wistful.

Really, my mother has been so motherly with me. She decided long ago that she would parent her children with discussion, instead of the dictatorship style her parents had used. Her mother had rarely expressed love with her. Because Pat-Pat had a long unspoken list of frustrations about what having four kids had prevented her from doing. Beneath the veneer of her life was anger, a whole lot of anger.

Later, before she died, it was if her Alzheimer's had softened her back, wiped away her memory, and given us her essence, a woman who cried and hugged us often. But in my childhood, she was not cuddly. She was a devoted grandmother who read me stories and laughed a big loud laugh. She praised me for doing my homework. In her presence, we always sensed that right and wrong were hard lines etched into concrete. She wore a gold cross around her neck. As a girl, I begged to watch her unscrew the small lid and open it to reveal the tiniest scroll and a piece of the Cross, the real Cross of Jesus.

I couldn't get over that.

"It's really the *real* Cross?" I would ask, and she laughed and told me yes as I inched closer and grazed my small hand against what looked like a grain of big sand.

"You can touch it," she would say, knowing that we all want to touch a part of ancient history.

He had been so wounded and so strong.

For all the supposed sins of the body (sex, sex, masturbating, and sex), there was so much Body in the Catholic Church despite most religions' distaste for the earthly body. We ate his body every Sunday. My mom and I would stand in church, holding hands, me a girl, she a woman, no inkling of the divine feminine, not yet at least.

What I am needing now is a sort of church.

My daughter is three months old.

Some days I don't know what is up or down.

I can't believe most women go back to full-time work at this point.

I don't know what is happening.

My body has fallen apart.

~

The week of my birthday, in July, I want to destroy everything. My arms shake, shake, shake, accumulated energy, want to windmill them, see what happens. My strong creature jaw could bite through anything. I want to destroy my marriage. I want to destroy my husband, my parents, my health, my skin, the salad staring back at me,

my hair, my dog, the fucking Oriental rug. I want to destroy myself.
I spot a pair of my balled-up socks and want to hurl them against
the wall. They are too soft. I need something hard. There is nothing
hard anywhere. I don't pause to wonder why the sudden surge. It came
unannounced this time. It didn't start with any person. The rage just
showed up. I want to disassociate from it, remove it from my system.
Not mine, not mine. I also justify its expression; of course I get to say
and do whatever I want. Don't hold me down. Don't silence me. Get
out of my way, everyone.

Somehow I don't want to destroy Eula. I thank the moon for keeping her safe. I don't feel safe from myself. At night, I thrash around
in bed. I haven't slept in weeks, months. I need to sleep. I can't sleep.

"When's the last time you meditated?" asks my mom.

"What kind of question is that?" I say.

"I want to destroy everything," I tell my counselor, Janice, over the
phone. She has known me and guided me on and off for eleven years,
watched me evolve with my fear. I'm a shit-pile now, though. She can
feel into most anything I am feeling, but she isn't a mother to a child
herself. How did I end up on the muddy opposite bank of a wide dark
river from her? She calls out to me from across the abyss. I can't hear
what she is saying. I stare at the moon again. It tells me Eula is here
for her own reasons, but also here to purify me.

"I know," I yell, "I've already figured that out."

A week later, blood.

My menses floods red out of me. Exactly a year ago, I bled for the
last time before conception. When night falls, I grip my chest and feel
a release, great tide flows away away away, and with it goes so much
of the rage. I know my body is not supposed to be bleeding yet, not
while nursing.

It's probably a sign of something bad.

But I don't care. I welcome the blood. I welcome coming back
into a cycle.

~

What I learn: In ancient Greece, people used menstrual blood to fertilize fields. Thor, the Norse god, reached enlightenment by bathing in a river of menstrual blood. In Celtic Britain, a king could become divine if he drank "red mead" from the fairy queen Mab. That women could bleed without dying was magical—not as much to women, who knew it as a monthly experience, but to men, who could not bleed this way. The Babylonian word *Sabbath* comes from *Sabat* and means "heart rest"—it was considered a day of rest for everyone while the goddess Ishtar was menstruating. It was a time to restore. It was a retreat. It is often known as a blood mystery or blood bonding. Women themselves often went away during menses, not because they were considered impure, as is often thought in modern conversation. The separation from everydayness was an honoring of how the womb sloughs blood—lets go of grief for the woman *and* her community. She would enter a place of supreme internal darkness, often in the company of other women, and use her body's wisdom to tend to the natural emotional upheaval that surfaces for any human.

I start to see an unexplored alchemy.

Most of my peers have grown up talking about the major inconvenience of periods. We even have birth control pills to eliminate bleeding altogether. I started to value my cycle in my late teens but never knew it could be a monthly flush and tool for deep release, for me, for others.

~

Okay, I must take real steps toward healing: more internal work, more kindness toward my mom, more self-care, and more sleep. Especially since I'm going back to part-time work in a month. Chris suggests that *adding* more pressure (or anything) may not be the best approach during this transition. I respond with apologies: "Thank you, babe, thank you. I'm sorry, I've felt so uncontrollable, I'm sorry for everything." But it does require more effort to get Eula to sleep so that we can sleep. I want to be done with "working hard" on naps and I've only just started. Some of my friends had major sleep issues with their children and have told me that the earlier you corral the nap thing the better. I've let my fear be my guide.

We cover her co-sleeper with a tight gray blanket for naps. It's the only way to darken the guesthouse completely during the day. My father teases that her bed looks like a sarcophagus. We have to hide the world from her, otherwise she finds a pattern—shadows, fan, window, blue checked blanket—and her eyes don't close. Still so much bouncing required. I do what new mothers do and make it a positive. She must simply be off-the-charts visual. She won't let any texture go by without a dialogue. Who wants a placid child anyway? I use the fact as currency to keep me functional. Every day I remind myself I've done well as a parent: shown her the dark green of a zucchini, smooched her belly a lot, laughed with her, held her against my breast, observed as best as I can.

When we go to our next Milk Bar gathering, I plan to ask about naps.

We never get to that conversation, though.

One woman mentions how her thighs rub together now.

"Me too," sighs another woman.

"Me too," sighs another woman from the hallway.

"I mean, whose thighs didn't rub together pre-birth?" I laugh.

But no one laughs.

They go back to tending babies and I choose to hear what I think their silence says but really doesn't: *Mine didn't, Mine didn't, Mine didn't.*

"Well, mine did," I say.

I have self-doubt around my legs. Have for a long stretch now. These days, they move like two logs. They keep me steady but barely hold up the heavy hammock between them. The only way to love my legs again is to let them out. They've been hidden. More love for my legs. More. My mom takes Eula for a few hours and I drive to Kohl's, where I never shop because I never shop and because everything is made by child laborers. I tell myself this is okay; right now, it's okay. My mission: shorts, maybe a skirt, though I'm not a skirt person. The mirrors must be slimming because I don't think my legs look that bad. I leave with $132 worth of shorts, and one skort.

~

Part of my "more" is making space to go within every single day.

It happens once a week.

For one, I imagine a huge heavy yoke fastened around my hips, like a skirt with metal hanging from it. It weighs my pelvis down. It is knotted thousands of times at my belly button. This yoke can represent whatever holds you down. My women hold me up, but these days I make the yoke my mother and her mother and her mother and her mother, the women. I pretend to stand on a dock. I start to undo the knots, one by one. My face heats up and tears flow freely. I let it happen and lower the yoke down, the whole carcass of it, the part that hangs on my sacrum. Then I lift it and walk toward my mother and her mother and her mother and her mother and lay it at their feet.

"This is yours," I say. "I don't need it anymore."

They don't respond.

They vanish. Where have they gone; where is the yoke? Suddenly I want it back, to swing it over my shoulder, so I don't lose them.

But, wait, pause, I feel light, consecrated. I dive off the dock backward into cool water and swim to an island. Alone. I am alone in the loneliness without my yoke. It's an awful sick necessary feeling. Maybe my mother can give the yoke back to her mother, who can give it back to her mother, until we reach original woman, who will bury it in the dark, dank, deep earth.

We women carry each other—whether we want to or not, whether we plan to or not. Our legs carry the pelvis and carry us across the earth. If we stacked pelvis upon pelvis upon pelvis, would it become a backbone? Everyone originates in the pelvis. Do you know that, Eula? You were an egg inside me, who was an egg inside Mare, who was an egg inside Pat-Pat.

~

My women friends are far-flung. My cousin Lauren, though, comes to visit. She will be part of me helping myself. She wants to meet *Eula the warrior goddess* (what she calls her) in person. When she steps through the airport door, she marches toward me like a queen—fresh from New York. She knows how to move.

"Ahhhhh," she says, and shakes her hands by her face, wipes the tears, and strokes Eula's cheek.

Eula is too much. Too much. This whole thing is too much.

"I know, Lo," I say. "It's crazy."

I grab her hand and we go.

Her hands are always warm, even hot. They've been that way since we were little.

Lauren dyed her hair black a few years ago. People take her more seriously this way, she says. She is the most glamorous person I know, a confidence in her body no one can even label, a size 10/12 like me. When men used to grab at her armpit hair in bars and call it sexy, she would shove them away. Almond eyes. Closets, I mean closets full of clothes. I fit my wardrobe in two drawers. She embodies some art of modern womanhood I chose not to learn from my mother. I help her troubleshoot how to take her trash out every week and how to believe in her deep self-worth. We once stood in front of a mirror at her father's lake house, both lean from summer and outdoors, me freckled, her tan, my hair short as a boy's, her hair long and blond, and we marveled at our different creature-ness.

Our fierceness is our sameness.

When Lauren leans over the bed, her long necklaces dangle out and Eula grabs for them. At dinner, my parents, Chris, and I can't stop laughing at Lauren's everything. She is still entertaining us—talks about the phrase "big-boned" and what does that really mean, that her bones are this big, just big around, like trees. We laugh so hard we think we might pee and I do pee right into my *Always* Extra-Long Pad with Wings. Later, when we are getting ready to sleep, she lifts her shirt and grabs the extra fat on her stomach. Squeezes it together. When she did that in front of her boyfriend and made talking sounds from her stomach, he scolded, "Never do that again." I grab my stomach with her and there we are, two women grabbing our stomachs, making them talk.

"What the hell," I say about her boyfriend.

Chris is laughing at us, at the whole thing, in the kitchen. I appreciate him siding with us. He is that sort of man, usually.

The next day, Lauren and I lie in bed on our backs, hold Eula above us, and pass her back and forth as she gurgles and smiles.

"I feel like we are fourteen and babysitting someone else's child," Lauren says.

"I feel the same way," I agree, and continue, "actually, sort of. It's very real. This girl has exploded my heart open. Words are stupid about it. No words for it. And there is the minor detail that I haven't slept since she was born."

"Oh gawd," Lauren says, calling up our grandmother's safe version of *Oh God*.

"Where did you come from?" Lauren says, cooing at Eula.

"Did you know Pat-Pat over there?"

We smile, wondering at the eternal reincarnation cycle.

Then, Lauren looks at me with wide eyes and looks back at Eula. "Are you Pat-Pat?"

~

The wheat fields have turned shocking white. This is how summer ends here. Green to gold to white and days shorten and air cools. That cooling of the air against brittle leaves reminds me of nausea, of what it felt like to be pregnant.

Our local hot springs can help me heal.

It's ten minutes down the road. Some people are turned away because it doesn't evoke the spiritual aspect of what we think of when we think of hot springs. I was repelled at first too: loud echoes of the indoor pool, crumbling edge of the outdoor pool, and a candy stand in the entrance. But I go at dawn, when few are there. Sweat in the wood sauna, plunge in the cold pool, and float in the outdoor pool beneath tall fir trees graced by nesting hawks.

The earth here in the American West produces hot blessed water.

It has helped others heal. It can help me heal.

More, yes, more.

Thank you, water.

My brother Alex comes to visit and I take him and my parents to the other hot springs, the open-air one farther away along the Madison River. I haven't properly introduced my mother to this new place. She uprooted her life. She has few friends here. She knows so little of the geography. I've been unable to be her guide and want that to change. My father doesn't require the same sort of settling into a place. He won't go in the water because he doesn't like hot water, but he'll come along. Chris cannot come because he is framing the house.

"You sure, babe?" I ask.

"I'm in the flow," he says down at the site, stacks of wood around him, three different measuring tapes in his tool belt. He smooches Eula and tells us to have fun. I watch his eyes and recognize how much he loses from everyday life by giving us the long-term gift of this house. Can that even change at this point? I don't know. This is the start of the middle of his trauma. We don't recognize it yet, and he won't have words for it until much later: the hurt of watching me hurt and then of me hurting him out of my hurt and of us hurting each other, the pressure of making our home with his hands, the stress of how to make our life and jobs sustainable. There will be a moment where he tells me he needs space for his own darkness and needs to trust I won't "just walk out." Then the cascade of moments when he understands he has been silent, with his parents and brother, with me, with himself. We talk to each other but cannot grasp what the other person feels right now. I talk to my friends about motherhood and womanhood most days. But his intimate conversations with men come at intervals, out of happenstance, at a dinner where people go around the table and answer a life question and he says something profound and his tears well up. He doesn't reach out. Not because of shame; just because it doesn't happen. Our focus with one another will shift then, but we aren't there yet. We aren't even close. I'm not even close. Right now, we fall into a hug, his tired body, my tired body, our family.

Surrounded by sagebrush and wetland, my mother slips into

translucent green water. It's an outdoor wooden communal tub. The way she folds the towel carefully around her reveals her reserved way, a way she's been as long as my life. She and Alex dunk their heads and arc back up to sun. A cold sprinkler sprays into the pool. Somewhere a flock of blackbirds balances on the fence. Somewhere other people, just a few, soak. Somewhere steam is rising.

My mom takes Eula while I go to change.

I emerge in my swimsuit. I'm chest out, like a rooster. Ready for water. Eula is smiling as my mother whooshes her in and out of the water, whoosh, whoosh, whoosh, this wise baby of mine, of ours. Once I'm in, once the hot water warms my thighs, my mother seems like a girl to me, and my ache for her is so strong I have to hold on to the concrete pool edge. I don't understand how we can both despise and love our mothers so deeply—as if they are nothing to us, as they are everything to us.

"Look at her feel it with her hands," I say, and lean my nose to hers. Eula touches the water, watches it drip from her fingers, watches it swallow her hand again. I don't remember when or how I learned to swim, only the knowledge of my mother nearby, reliable, present, with her children in cool pools in hot tropical places.

Alex is doing his Alex thing, face up to the sun, deep breathing.

I notice people looking at him. They are wondering. They always wonder whether he's famous, which he's not, at least not yet, he would say. He looks famous with his tall tan body and black-rim glasses. So many people in my mother's family look famous. My mother did when she was young, but she didn't know it.

I have never looked famous.

I don't want to look famous to others. I want to feel famous to myself. They might be the same thing. I am starting to understand that looking famous comes from feeling famous, which comes from inhabiting a pose, which comes from honoring yourself, which comes from loving your body, which comes from accepting that the sun is delighted to shine on your own holy face.

~

Eula is four months old and I am going back to work. It's my own schedule, a few mornings or afternoons a week. Teaching writing workshops and helping individuals find voice is my true vocation. I don't dread it. I am lucky. The hardware of my transition is in place: breast pump works; two glass bottles purchased; child did not, thank goodness, reject the plastic nipple.

But what am I really prepared for here?

Welcome back to the public. Put some clothes on. I've forgotten so many real-life details. The medical bills from Eula's birth have started to arrive. We've stacked them in a pile near the sink. They flash at me like strobe lights. At least we'll meet our high deductible. Maybe we should go see all the doctors we don't really need to see just to take advantage of this situation: get my moles and freckles checked, go to a podiatrist for that foot pain, ask an eye doctor about that spot in my eye. Really, though, none of those should be extraneous visits. Blue Cross Blue Shield covers so little, never covers much for any-one, especially women, especially the self-employed. Every medical expense we have, with the exception of one yearly doctor checkup, is out-of-pocket for us. No small co-pays. Nothing "free." We are, sadly, a common situation in our country. Here's where I check my privilege, again—because I did not grow up poor, because I did go to college, because I am white, because if I was desperate for one hundred dollars to pay a bill, I could borrow it from someone in my support system. And I can trade with Holcomb: my writing help for her doctoring. We will need to ask the hospital for a payment plan. It's the only way. But first start by being consistent about doing your pelvic-floor exer-cises. My mind is a foot soldier with me—*do them, do them*—when all I want to do is lie on the couch. Even though I've vowed off surgery. The push and pull. As Pat-Pat used to say, you can't help someone who isn't trying to help herself.

I am trying, but I get deflated.

I also don't know what's happening in the world. Haven't been able to follow the news. The other day in town, I saw an older woman friend for the first time since Eula's birth. She asked how I was. I seem normal to everyone because I'm good at appearing normal. With my friendly smile, I told her about incontinence.

"We all pee on ourselves, all us mothers," she said. "Welcome to the club."

I think she means she pees a little when she sneezes, not gushes urine when she simply walks downhill. But here is what I wanted to say: I don't want to be in this club. Why are you okay with this club? Why are so many women okay with this? Why are they quiet about it? What if men were the ones who suffered loss of urine control after pushing the next generation of humans into the world? Would we have federally funded programs to alleviate the problem?

By noon, I need to be functional and presentable for a client. That means I need to brush my hair and tone down the viper. She is stomping around the house. Look at her bat at her husband's dirty socks. Look at her want to run away. Look at her know she can't because she would never leave her daughter. Look at her feel trapped. Look at her slam the fridge door. Look at her eat half a quesadilla and then pitch it in disgust. Look at her dog watch her, unsure of what is happening. Look at her pick up her daughter and walk next door to ask her mother to please come over because she needs to shower and doesn't think she can do it while managing her baby today. Look at her stoop in shame at being dependent. Look at her cry in the shower. Look at the way her face opens and sustains a silent scream.

When I emerge from the shower, the air is fresh. Out the window, yellow leaves flutter on trees. My mother and Eula are reading *The Runaway Bunny*, one of my childhood favorites. They glance up at me and both smile with big kind blue eyes.

~

Our sleep ritual of shades drawn and ocean sounds is a hardcore routine now. I wonder if the lack of light is part of what is getting to me. I don't know whether this feeling is a normal part of new motherhood or living near my parents or trying to heal or what. When we want light, Chris and I sneak into the tiny bathroom to eat dinner and talk. We've had sex here, in the light, twice. Unlike many of my mama friends, I'm not repelled by it. Somehow my body hungers for it more. But something has recently changed—a disassociation with men, like they, like he, is foreign to me, like I get what I need and then detach.

With our bowls of food, we sit in the bathtub or on the toilet lid.

"Babe," I say to Chris, "I think I'm grieving about my body." I'm proud of having said it with my sadness instead of my rage.

"Okay," he says, and that's it. He doesn't ask me about what. I don't know how to respond to his non-responses. He has never been so inadequate to me as he is these days. We are far from the days when he used to ride his bike down a dark country road just to kiss me good night before going back to study for a chemistry test, when we wrote poetic missives to one another on recycled paper, when we stitched pillows and pressed leaves into books, when he would massage my feet and I would stroke his head. When did we become these jaded people? I never thought we would follow the standard trajectory of what society tells us happens to new parents. Like he requested, I try to show him my sadness instead of anger but it doesn't matter. I know this isn't his fault. He is in the process of becoming a father, along with the pressure of building our home, tired hands, tired body, tired soul, all day on a roof. But I want to blame him. I want to blame someone for how I feel, who I have become, and what is happening, even though I can't put a name to what is happening.

I'm not depressed.

I'm fractured.

I'm mad.

~

More nature. More movement. This will help. My mother and I go walking, down the dirt driveway and onto the dirt road with Eula sleeping in a stroller meant for places like this, wheels as big as wagon wheels. An overcast September sky floats over us, thick and low and gray in the west. We walk toward it. Here is my mother, so willing always. When I bled through my pad as breast milk dripped down my chest, she laughed, "Well, this is motherhood," and suddenly, holding my Eula, I was aware of being part of a vast underground network. I wanted to stop mothers on the street and ask, "You do this too?"

We pass by the yellow farmhouse and walk toward a haystack. The sky turns black.

"Let's turn around; look at that squall line," she says. *Squall line* sounds like something my father, the man of sailboats, the son of people of sailboats, would say.

"No, let's push it," I reply.

A few minutes later, the dark sky wakes up. It comes at us fast, wisps of black reaching for the white sky, consuming it. The white sky has no chance.

"Let's go," I say.

Now we are running.

But you can't run away from this. You are in it. The stroller bumps along as my feet pound on dirt, as my vagina falls out, as my pelvis absorbs the mass of me. Go, go, go. Black clouds, you are pure. Black clouds, you are fast. We run from what could become heavy hurtful hail. But we laugh, we are laughing so hard that pee runs down my legs into the earth.

"Here comes the wind," she shouts with her arms up in the air, an openness from her mouth. I haven't seen my mother like this before, so aware and amazed by nature. She stops, heaving breath. So I stop. She says, "Keep going, I'll catch up." I don't keep going. We stand together and wind whips through the cottonwoods. We start to run again. We have two hundred yards to go. We are running. Don't let a tree branch fall because that could actually kill us. Keep the hail away for a few more minutes. Keep the dark from swallowing us.

The gravel crunches under our feet.

Women have always known how to run.

Women have always been in conversation with the dark.

I had no idea that I had no idea about my mother.

I had no idea how hungry I would become to align with her and away from man.

"Almost there," we shout together, as wind and cold and black push at our backs.

And this is it. We live in the storm, and we are laughing and we are moving away from it, but we are okay in it too. We are okay. Eula wakes and starts to hum along with the storm. As we bump and run home, she recognizes its blackness, its wildness as kin.

~

Eula, at five months old, wakes only twice one night—this feels like a miracle. We've been doing the "flip and shush," and she prefers sleeping on her belly. Maybe that has helped. A gray dawn filters though windows. I am so electrified by the possibility of consistent sleep I can't actually sleep. I try to do pelvic-floor exercises but the reality exhausts me. Chris reaches over to me, acknowledges we've actually slept some. We start to rub each other, to rub up against each other, and maybe this is what happens with the balm of sleep. Bru feels the calm wash over him and inches closer to our bed, crawls in with us. We are limbs over limbs over limbs over limbs and nothing has ever been so cozy. We stare at Eula and whisper that maybe this is a new phase. Maybe we'll have to wake only a few times each night from now on, or maybe not wake at all. Maybe this is the beginning of ease. But maybe it's not and I should know better. I should know that nothing is permanent. I should go with whatever flow. I should know that she'll hit her next growth spurt and she'll be awake and uncomfortable and then so will I because that is what we do, isn't it, help each other grow? Because though growing is necessary, growing is hard.

~

These days my mood veers into a ditch with the slightest gust of wind. Is this who I am, have always been? Where is the good me? She expects consistency from herself. The other me's know consistency is a fallacy. Nothing in nature and humanity is consistent and there's a reason for that. Maslow's hierarchy of needs pyramid doesn't occur to me yet. Without physiological basics—sleep, excretion, homeostasis, breathing, food, shelter—a person can't function well in any other parts of life or relationships. I'm solid, though. I'm supported. But the loss of urinary continence has wiped out all other possibilities in my life and made the smallest everyday tasks feel enormous. Even I don't fully admit to the impact of it. I tell myself to just get over it, get myself to the grocery store, buy food, take care, deal with the pee pads, deal with living out of a duffel bag, deal with not knowing where my clothes are, serve my daughter and mend my mood.

I don't dare wonder anymore what it would feel like to slip on some sexy underwear without a pad and walk around town with my daughter on my hip without any discomfort or pressure on my pelvis.

I don't dare.

Instead, the upset surfaces in other ways. When the viper awakens within me, I cannot control my rapid escalation. Walk away. Take a breath. Come back later. Write it down instead. None of that works yet. None of that shifts my surge, my urge to say it *now* and say it true.

One afternoon, something in me breaks.

"We may not be able to have an overhang on our roof," Chris says in a flat voice.

"Okay, but should we pause to consider that? How does that affect where the snow falls?"

"It's more work for me to put an overhang on."

"Okay."

I don't know how to say what I need to say. He won't look me in the eye. He gathers his pile of graph papers and starts to pour a coffee. I move toward a corner to rub my face, hand on my chest, slow yourself down, Molly, slow yourself down.

"Babe," I say, "I just think we should pause. That's a big decision."

That is not what he wants to hear. He wants a shortcut. He wants a break. I understand and I don't understand. He makes no sign that he's heard me. He chooses not to hear me. The cement wall between us has no fissures for any light.

"Babe," I repeat.

"Hey, Chris," I say as he starts to walk toward the door.

My whole body starts to shake.

"Listen to me," I shout.

I put Eula down. He is not listening. He is not listening.

I grab a pile of laundry and throw it at him. Most of it floats halfway between us, lands with a gentle thud on the ground. Someone starts to scream and I don't realize it's me until he has picked up Eula and they are out the door, with our cowering dog. They are fleeing because they must. My. Beloved. Family. I fall on the bed and punch it, punch the hell out of it, my arms working hard, until my sobs calm, until I am limp, a limp woman. Something is wrong with this limp woman. She cannot stop the sentences now. The thoughts. They come fast.

Where is the strong laboring woman who was here, right on this bed?

Where is she?

She was in control of the out of control.

I refuse to believe this is only lack of sleep. Something is wrong with me. Will people in the grocery store stop calling Eula serious? She isn't serious. She's an observer. She doesn't smile unless she wants to. I tell her, "You are free, I take responsibility for my emotions, these toxic emotions, you are free of them." I hope she believes me. I can't stop crying in the shower. If she sees me cry, I explain I'm sad but it's okay. People get sad sometimes, Eula. People get angry sometimes, Eula. It's normal. But this, this right now, doesn't feel normal.

~

I stand in my mother's red-floored kitchen and hear myself complain. Eula only had a twenty-minute nap. I'm bleeding again. All the other nursing mamas don't have their menses back yet. I wanted to be able to be a mother who hiked every day with her daughter.

My daughter, in my arms, watches me say it all.

"And now . . . she's imprinting on me," I sigh. "This is all she knows of me. Weak pregnant woman. Weak new mother. Weak all around. I want to be the mom who is out and about."

"Don't go there. You can't worry about that. Just let that go," says my mom. "You are not a weak mother. You have been on walks in the woods with Eula. You are an amazing mom. You laugh with her all the time. You pay close attention to her. She will grow up feeling seen by you, Moll. But I am concerned about *you*. I knew there was a reason I needed to be here this fall."

Her words wash down the shore from me.

"I just have no time to sit down," I say.

"I know," my mom agrees. "I never sat down either. And when I did, I felt guilty."

"*God*," I growl, "why is that the case for so many women? Chris takes her for half an hour in the morning and I feel bad about it, like I shouldn't burden him. I thought I'd trained myself out of that old model."

"I know."

This phenomenon exasperates me. I'm sure Pat-Pat conversed with that guilt; perhaps every woman in my lineage, in most lineages, has wrestled with some form of it.

Later that night, I sit on the bathtub's edge and explain to Chris.

"Eula only knows me as ill Mom, as angry person; that's so sad for her."

"Babe, that isn't true at all. That's just another arm of your guilt. Let it go."

He names it for me, just as my mom did.

He doesn't require me to feel guilty. He never has.

Eula and I play harmonica. We hold on to it together. She blows into one side while I do the other. This makes us laugh and laugh. We sing songs about listening for birds and how Papa is on the roof, and the only line I can come up with about me is that Mama is dressed in red.

~

My mother makes both of these comments to me in one day:

One: "Molly, I realize language is important to you. What you said about the word *pretty* is true. It can limit a girl's understanding of herself." She holds her hand out to me. This validation feels like sweet syrup in my system. "And," she adds, "you are such a good mom for knowing that, and being mindful about it." I re-explain that *pretty* isn't a bad word, let's just not make it the first and only word people use with her. It's so often the *one* word anyone uses for a girl—and a girl is so many other adjectives besides *pretty*. I don't want to coddle my daughter or shield her from common language, but it is an act of intelligence to be awake to it.

Two: "I don't want Eula to look like a pauper when we go to Chicago. Polka dots and stripes don't go together." I stare at my baby in her polka dots and stripes and tell my mother I don't care about what goes together. She grumbles and walks into the kitchen to chop vegetables. I fume on the chair, stroking my daughter and telepathically communicating to her that she is perfect as is. I don't want her to feel the family obsession with pleasing others through clothes. Then, as I get up to leave, my mother adds, "Sheesh, we're also going to have to spend some time getting *your* clothes together for the trip." I know she is referencing the huge and elaborate party my uncle and aunt host—that she thinks I never have the right sort of dress or slacks. "Mom, I'm thirty-four years old. I can dress my own body," I say, and I let the screen door slam behind me.

We wax and wane.

My mother might utter two incongruous statements in a day.

But I am capable of twenty.

~

Here we go again. Control the mother. At early November, Eula gets sick for the first time, with a hoarse cough. It sounds like whooping cough. I become a dragon trolling through the shallow ocean looking for someone to blame. I find Chris but he is also sick, passed out on our bed. My mother appears like a beacon. She can handle anything. She also has a cough, after all.

"Do you think you caught this cough somewhere?"

"Molly, it may not be the same thing," she says.

"*Someone* brought it into the home."

"Fine, if you are looking for someone to blame, blame me," she huffs back, and walks out.

I'm scared. I'm scared something is really wrong with Eula. I lash out because the fear wants to burst out of my chest. I just need to say,

"I'm scared, Mom," and be the me who is normally calm when other people are sick. But this is not *other people*; this is my child; this is the first time I've seen her body struggle. If I want Eula to grow into a woman who forgives herself, then I must become a woman who forgives myself. It's okay you made a mistake. It's okay you lashed out. You can set a goal to be different next time. My mom is the one who tells me I was so hard on myself as a child. She didn't know what to do about it. She would pull me aside and say, "You don't have to be so hard on yourself, honey." Nothing helped. She decided I was made that way. Some people are made that way.

Once Eula recovers, my mother commiserates.

"I remember the first time you were sick. You woke up like a wet rag."

"Really?"

"Yeah, that was scary."

"What was I sick with?"

"I don't remember," she says.

"How did I recover?"

"You always recovered fast."

~

It's been six months. Shouldn't I be rising out of the ashes of a hard pregnancy and complicated birth by now? My body moves through molasses these days. I am so very tired. After Eula has fallen asleep, I crawl away from sitting to standing and eventually toward the bathroom, willing my toes not to crack. Shut the fuck up, toes. She can hear that imperceptible sound of me, past the ocean waves, past Bru snoring, past Chris coughing, she hears my toes, because she knows it as me and I have boobs full of milk and I'm her mama. It could be a tender memory. But my exhaustion makes it not so. When she wakes at night now, I become a violent whale in bed, one who slaps the covers over her husband. I want to be sure he knows I am awake—again. How will I ever dance or cartwheel with her? My prolapse is worse. My incontinence is the same. Put a diaper on Eula, put a pad on myself. Every day. Maybe we'll potty train together one day.

One morning I wake up and cannot move my body from bed.

Eula rests nearby in her co-sleeper. I don't know how I will reach her.

"I'm so tired," I call out to Chris, and I start to cry. "I feel like I can't move." He continues to bustle around in the kitchen; he's ignoring me; he's over and done with my issues.

"Babe," I say, "I need help, please help me."

"Babe," I say, and my cry morphs to a roar, ". . . please."

But he walks out the wooden door without a word.

The shock waves crash into me. What do I do now? How do I reach my baby? I roll over to her and pull her toward me, toward our full day in bed. My tears stop because she gazes up at me. Over the phone, Holcomb speculates it might be thyroid, and she calls in a few blood tests.

So it is.

Postpartum thyroiditis. On the same day, our pup gets diagnosed with the same thyroid issue. He watched me vomit all through pregnancy and has been beside me during the entire transition, this sensitive dear animal of ours. I stroke him, hold his snout, my eyes to his eyes, and say, "You don't have to take this on, you don't."

We go together to pick up our pills.

I've never been a pill person. Now I have to be. I put this medication and my herbs in an empty glass spice jar to make them appear exotic and stunning. It will help me take them.

This diagnosis is not uncommon for new mamas; however, my numbers teeter on the edge of an autoimmune disease. Not there yet, though. This is good. Holcomb says she's impressed I've been able to teach, take care of Eula, and function in general. This information becomes my sword. See, I want to tell everyone, especially Chris. See. I wasn't making it up. This is real. It's scientific. I am not so crazy. Beneath the gratification is more rage. My body is officially broken. I pee on myself *and* my thyroid doesn't work. I might feel sluggish and heavy my entire life. Great. To jump-start and heal my thyroid, I need to exercise. But when I exercise, pee pours out of me. It's an impossible cycle.

There is no out.

There is a grander story at work.

I cannot yet make the link now.

Just be grateful you have a healthy daughter. You aren't dying. Don't complain.

~

What I learn: The emotional causes for hypothyroidism are both res-onant and not. I do not feel like an unexpressed woman. Perhaps my good-girl childhood contributed to part of that, but not much. I've never not shared what I think—what I *feel*, though, is debatable and based on my audience. Holcomb mentioned thyroid disease is often associated with long periods of mild depression, meaning the depression is actually caused by the thyroid problem. Someone can be misdiagnosed very easily. I don't know how to parse the physical ver-sus the mental. They are one. I'm responsible for all of it. In Chinese medicine, hypothyroidism is considered an imbalance, a deficiency of yang masculine energy: no get up and go, a "giving up" sensation. The giving up is accurate. If Eula didn't need my care, I would lie facedown on the muddy earth all day. Not my inherent way. My tem-perament has always been more masculine. Maybe the feminine yin energy is trying to bloom in me—what a way to do it, though. They say bladder problems indicate fear and suppressed anger. My body has called the rage up. It is not a symptom. It's old. It's the deeper unex-pressed I thought I didn't have.

~

Maybe our oldest female story starts in the pelvis and moves out the throat. My oldest female story also comes from the family created by my maternal grandmother. We go to her homeland, Chicago, for Thanksgiving, where everyone born of Pat-Pat gathers. My old wounds usually crawl out of holes in this setting, despite the inclu-siveness—true, maybe, of all childhood places.

My aunt and uncle throw a massive party every November. It brings together families who raised their now college-attending kids together. It's a way to recapture all they've shared as friends over the years. Lauren and her younger sisters, my cousins, pose in mirrors and swap dresses and draw on makeup. It's a ritual. It's happened for years. They laugh and dance. They'd rather be in pajamas but they have to dress up because three hundred people are downstairs waiting to see them, and their friends, the other young adults at the fresh start of their lives. Though they invite me to be part of it, I do not consider myself *of* that element. I feel like the fat cousin and usually end up crying in a closet alone.

This time must be different.

There will be no crying in closets.

I have to be strong for Eula. She will watch my every move and learn from it. Chris, my steady background in these moments, knows the history and tells me it'll be great. The thyroid news has either hardened or loosened me because I wear my black lace tango dress and walk around detached and unaffected. People buzz around and call me pretty and I choose not to be my usual offended when someone says with surprise, "Whoa, you are beautiful."

When my brothers comment, "Oooo, lace," I don't attack by telling them I do actually own some feminine items. They often tease me about my clothes and body. They mean it as a point of loving connection but it's still a tease. The world teases women, not men, never men, about clothes and body. Do they know they are cogs in this system? With Eula in my arms, I wonder whether I've crossed, or half crossed, the wet valley of this particular beauty sadness.

Is this what progress feels like?

When the party ends, when the mass of people have left, my cousins and aunt hop up to dance on the granite kitchen counter in short dresses. Everyone can finally relax and be done with small talk. Eula squeals with delight at all the action, and I tell myself it's okay, it's okay, it's okay. One day that can be me, if I want it. It is me in other settings with other people. But I don't need to want it here. My mom isn't up there. She's across the room, watching them, just like me, with red wine glass in hand, smiling but with a defeated look. I can feel her feeling. The cord between us thickens brown and strong. We are aligned here, in some way—women who are shy, who don't fully know how to express our sensuality in public, who feel out of our knowing in this moment of hotness.

~

When we return to December snow, I decide, again, to take seriously the act of self-care. Another vow of mine; Chris often says if there's one thing I do always and without fail, it's make plans and intentions. There are no longer huge unknowns. My health information has been gathered. Now the data and diagnosis computes out to give me a place to start from.

I can track my body and mind.

I can converse with my cells.

Meanwhile, I feed Eula gorgeous foods—pumpkin, avocado, and blackberries. These colors. We sit and *mmmmm* together and she, turns out, is a child who loves the sensual part of food. She rejects nothing. She wants to try everything. Watching her reminds me I am inherently that way too.

One afternoon, I cook carrots and we eat them together. I pretend to be introducing us both to this new food. We talk about it. The sweetness, the deep orange, how this vegetable grew in the earth, sent its taproot down. By the end, we are both covered in carrot and nourished. I want to believe I can keep this up. I want to believe a carrot can hold my attention. I want to believe I will choose a carrot over cookies. Cookies aren't bad. But I choose them often to hurt myself and to prove something to some people who aren't even listening anyway.

"Why does food matter so much to you?" a friend asks.

It's what my body is made of—colors and textures. I love food the way I love clothing the way I love all the things I've chosen to reject in the name of becoming a different sort of female. I want to care for myself the way I care for my daughter.

Eula starts to crawl.

I prance around her as she moves along the rug. She stops, starts, looks up at me, grins, chooses a direction to go, and then goes. Her world is exploding right now, right at this instant. Selfhood. Agency. The choice to grab her cow stuffed animal over the others. In a few days, I know my daughter better than I ever have—her preferences, decisions.

"Welcome to the world of locomotion," I say.

She grins again.

I dance to make her laugh and launch myself into a cartwheel. It sort of works, only air sucks into my vagina and then leaves it with a farting noise. No matter. My daughter is moving. This week, her movement journey has begun: walking, dancing, running, hugging, lovemaking, squatting, jumping, there is so much for a body to do.

There is so much for a body to do.

There is so much for a body to explore.

Remember this, I tell myself.

~

At night, I smell the milk of us, watch Eula's hands twitch as moon-light comes through the window and feel a vast freedom to craft my own relationship with my daughter, as we choose. My love for her has expanded into something far beyond the animal love of protection. This is now relational love. I would die if she died.

I'm sure of it.

"My love for her is so intense it hurts," I tell Chris.

"Me too," he says, and slips his hand in mine.

Beyond the house walls, birds sleep in the dark at 6 a.m. We pull Eula into our bed for snuggles. Not yet time for wake-up. Though, can it be? She has slept through the night. I told Chris she would on the eve of her turning eight months old. I just knew it. I am learning who my daughter is. We can predict each other's moves. And so she has. She pulls my hair and yanks on Chris's nose and tries to escape our blockage to get to the power cord nearby. We groan our love to her.

She finds the concrete wall by our heads with its little holes and marks.

"Ohhh, ooooo, ahhhh," she gurgles.

Her fingers explore the contours because it could be a moonscape.

That's when, in my attempt to keep one eye open and on her, I notice a smudge of almond butter on the conduit. I sit up. Leftover from labor, from those crackers I ate when my uterus contracted down, to hug Eula, to prepare her for her birth. That laboring woman was *me*. She has left a remnant of herself, an offering: here, take it, remember yourself. This is the woman I must remind myself of. She was in flow. She was not fearful. She let her body do what it needed to do. She knew how to fly and moan and hum to move her baby, and her own self, into the world.

I must call her up within me again.

~

Some days, a metal wrecking ball lands on my chest. It doesn't warn me of its approach. My arms are not steely enough to remove it. We wake up to a silent land, so much snow tree boughs hang full and low, almost to the ground. A predominant thought pokes at me: *I need my own house in order to heal.* I cannot heal in the chaos of duffel bags and storage and mostly absent husband and overstaying.

Heavy wrecking ball.

The plan had always been to move out of my parents' guesthouse in November. They want to use it as a rental. Our house was supposed to be finished by now. But houses are never done on schedule. Especially a house built by one man who is also co-parenting his daughter. But it's a first-world problem and it was our choice.

So get over it.

My mom sweeps off her own porch and calls me. The men are gone for a week, on separate work trips. Our driveway will be impassable until the plow comes, today, tomorrow, or a few days after that. But our path between houses needs to be shoveled today. If we don't, it will turn to ice and the whole winter will become a slip hazard. I tried to shovel once and it, just like the act of splitting wood, damaged my prolapse further. But she also has a prolapse.

"I can shovel," she says, like the elder of the village.

"Well, I can try too," I say, and mean it.

"No, you stay there with Eula," she commands.

We women of this lineage lift heavy objects. My mother never needed a man to help her haul groceries, bags of soil, huge clay pots, anything. I once slid canoes atop cars by myself, carried fifty pounds of apples up and down ladders, hurled a backpack onto my back and hauled it up steep mountains.

We know how to labor with our hands and arms and legs.

I once knew how.

Heavy wrecking ball.

Right when Eula finally descends into her nap, right as her eyelids start to flicker, right as I levitate away from her, breathless and relieved for a break from holding it together for my daughter, my mother busts through the door. She wears a black balaclava, heavy jacket, has a shovel in hand; steam envelopes her, she puffs toward me, toward us, and Bru pants at her heels.

"It's me," she says with the exuberance of a girl.

I should add to her joy but a scowl comes out of me because now Eula is awake and it will take me another hour to get her down and this makes my skin crawl, makes me question what I'm doing as a mother, and that's when I see the shift, how I have, in one scowl, tamped out my mother's light. She turns and scuttles out the door.

Why do I do this?

How do I do this?

Heavy fucking wrecking ball.

She helps me and I hurt her.

I want to own my violence. I want to own my violence toward women, my mother, myself. Every human has grown up in collective waters that perpetuate this violence toward women. We all do it, whether we know it or not. On some level, we are all misogynists. When I feel disgust toward my mother it is my disgust toward myself.

I am violent.

I am tender.

These coexist in me.

As I shush and rock Eula, the prayers bellow out of me.

I cannot be this angry woman with my mother.

I cannot be this angry woman with my daughter.

Please help me find the other part of me; where is the good part?

~

For our Christmas tree, I find an aspen branch and tuck it between two chairs. The only ornaments on it are from my female linage— the art deco orange-and-silver star from my great-grandmother Anne, the Japanese cloth balls from Pat-Pat, the painted eggs my mother bought in the Czech Republic. I put the red-and-aqua wooden giraffe from Mexico at the base. It sends Eula into paroxysms: part crying, part elation. She calms herself and then reaches out a hand to softly stroke it. This girl has a gentle touch.

Our tree is sparse.

It speaks to me.

I regret again how I have or have not treated my mom.

We sit in the cabin. She cuts pineapples for pineapple upside-down cake and chitters and chatters about something that doesn't interest the men and normally wouldn't interest me, but now I am on her side. I want to pull her toward me and say, "Let's be wacky together. We are wise." But I don't make any moves. I am too shy. I stand across the kitchen and inhale pineapple smell and know I'm going to be devastated when she dies and I will remember this moment and wish I had told her then, now, how remarkable she is.

~

What I learn: Rage is a circuit that starts in my pelvis and moves out two openings: my urethra or my throat. No wonder the screams, the urine. It is mine. It is also part of a greater current of all women: women like me, women of other races, cultures, languages, and terrain. It is our push back toward the institutional violence we've grown up in. It spews outward in response to patriarchy. If I am angry, women of color must feel it a hundred thousand–fold. We have un-similar experiences held in the similar container of femaleness. Beneath it all, for all women, is grief. Can you hear the wail? *We have a voice too. Our body is sacred. Do not defile it. We have been unseen, disrespected, shut down. Leave us alone.* But the strangest indoctrination happens. Rage also turns inward toward each other: violence from women toward women. Who does she think she is? Look at her. We inhabit the system that breaks us. I have directed my own violence toward my mother, the woman who made me. It's an easy and safe anger. It stands in for what we've been taught—violence toward self and our own female body.

~

As I grow in and out of myself, Eula grows toward movement. To nurse, she now sits up on my knee, switches from left to right breast and takes ownership of which one she wants when. Then she tries to scrape freckles off my face. In the bath, she holds on to my nipples and leans way way back.

"Easy, there," I say, and we laugh.

Eula yanks up on Pat-Pat's old wooden hibachi, a Japanese portable cooking apparatus. On the carpet, she practices her pull-ups with a huge smile of pride, one so big her cheeks make a square of her face. My mother has used the hibachi as a coffee table. It's been a central part of every home of ours, dark and oiled and familiar. This is to watch an ancient her-story for me.

My daughter can move now. With eyes and hand gestures, she communicates what she needs. The world has opened for her. Any fuss Eula had seems to have evaporated. I don't know whether it was her fuss or mine. She was just a baby getting used to being in a body. I am just a woman getting used to being in a body.

I beg the sky and moon to please take my grief away. If my future is as a young incontinent woman with a prolapse and a slow thyroid, well, so be it. One friend warns me not to accept it. Don't accept it. Don't stop trying to heal. But it is so much effort to heal. It doesn't matter, she says. Don't stop trying.

One afternoon, as Eula naps, I pour hot water over dandelion tea, kneel near the fire, and take stock. I go back to *my biography is my biology*. What have I received and what can I now release?

The fire flickers back.

It has no answers.

I do, though.

Undo a contract I made long ago with my body.

Became Aware of Her Blood

As my body careened toward breasts, hips, and menstruation, the world started to tilt, and continued to tilt, until everything turned sideways and stayed there. Some girls practiced a sway-walk or gathered in clusters on the concrete courtyard at school to giggle at boys. I still ran with gunpowder under my feet. We lived in Mexico City now. My friends had grown tall or round or stocky and I had not—that small unimportant fact afforded me a huge unspoken privilege in our sisterhood of nine-year-olds. They begged to sit next to me on the bus and wanted my opinion on whether to wear our school uniform green sweatshirts around the waist high or low on hips few of us had yet. They carried me everywhere, and in my smallness I became the biggest thing. When I scampered up a tree, they watched, waiting for me to come down. It was the last time I would be the one who laughs the loudest because everyone is, and always has been, watching her.

Some force had boarded me onto the silver-bullet train.

I would enter the land of womanhood well-placed.

When a friend snuck me into the backroom of her plant-filled house to watch a forbidden romance film, she told me it made her feel tingly down there. "Down where?" I asked, and leaned back into a beanbag. *"There,"* she pointed. I had never considered my *down there* until, a few weeks later, I crashed my bike and my legs scissored the sewer grate and a whack so intense woke me up to it.

This place, this new place, what was this place, what was it for?
My mother hadn't told me anything about it.

I would be small for a while longer, and it would be easy to say the period of smallness seeded a confidence in me. But my sureness came from being a first child and a girl who demanded the ear of her parents and got it. My family called me Queen Bee, a name meant as a compliment or dig, depending on the circumstance. When my mother wanted to spend all day at the market, I could convince her out of it. My brothers sat wide-eyed and accepted my monologues on the right way to be. "You can't pull a fast one over Molly," my father told people. This differentiated me from my mother. She could bargain hard with rug sellers and stand up like a *toro* for her kids, but some societal framework had weakened her position within our family system. Whenever she wanted to impart a wisdom or opinion to us, her voice got louder and louder and louder until we rolled our eyes and eventually a panic washed over her face, where am I, what do I say now, what was my point, what do I actually mean? I could speak in whispers and get the attention of my family.

This gave me power over my graceful mother.

It would mold us like a river molds two sides of a riverbank.

I was nine, ten, eleven.

Whenever she took me to a department store to shop for clothes, I would drag behind her, annoyed at the fluorescent lights and the gentle way she browsed for sale items. My arm would grab hers and say let's go. Just a minute. I couldn't wait a minute. Don't make me try this on. I don't care if it's made from good linen. I am not a peacock. She would give up on me—and sharing her useful tip that it was best to buy a few good-quality items instead of many cheaply made ones—and move on to herself. But I don't want to wait for you to decide that's the right dress for the upcoming wedding. As we drove home, with a bag of natural-colored clothing for me, I told my mother that when I was a woman I was not going to waste my time with shopping.

She never fought back.

She held her tongue and didn't slap me with the reality that if you want clothes, you need to shop.

She was usually kind and let me air my proclamations.

The suggestions, though, about my appearance had begun to accumulate—maybe that skirt instead of the other one, maybe a braid instead of hair down. Did I have to look a certain way, and for whom? In the folds of my heart, a disappointment had lodged. My beloved strong mother was suddenly focused on instructing me to keep my legs crossed, my hair combed, my intensity in check. There must be other ways to become a woman. I didn't see them around me. The word *feminine*, in my world, meant to be demure and accommodating to everyone but yourself. It made me want to throw punches. Yet, every year, we watched *Miss America* together, curled up on the couch. Because it was an event just for us, separate from the men in our family, I luxuriated in it. My mom would stroke my forehead as we talked over which woman was the best woman. The subtext of what we were doing was beyond both of us. Of course, we also watched *Road to Avonlea*, a quaint show about a rural town in early 1900s Canada with as much interest, as much pleasure.

Regardless, shards of glass had begun to poke up through the surface.

On a walk around the dusty ancient pyramids of Mexico, a familiar outing for our family, I took my first confused step away from my mother. Moon. Sun. I scampered up and down crumbled steps and then ran back to join my clan and hold my mother's hand. As my father and brothers walked ahead of us, down a wide passageway of time, I studied the shape of my father's legs.

I knew my legs were his legs.

"I'm glad I have Dad's legs instead of yours," I said to my mother.

"Oh?" she said.

"Yeah, definitely."

I knew I was hurting her.

I wanted to hurt her and I didn't know why.

Lauren and I had begun to push our own edges without knowing why either. We performed a provocative dance for our entire family on the green lawn of my grandparents' suburban condo in Illinois. She actually knew how to move. I followed along because the urge to be subversive had lit within me. Our grandmother Pat-Pat smiled and said nothing from behind her dual-tone sunglasses. Goodness. Goodness gracious, Catholic girls. She had always thought me, the straight-A student, smart and sensible and good. With her praise, a warm feeling bloomed in me. My intellect must be special. She didn't "Lord over" me the same way she did my mother.

My mother—smashed between the two fierce bookends of us—was more of a feeler, less apt to bite anyone who came toward her. How could I be both good and bad? The *good* label started to grate on me as soon as I could name it. I didn't feel like a good girl when I noticed the boys (and men) were never asked to do dishes. Lauren and I huddled in a corner to make a plan.

"Okay, we have an announcement," we called out. We would not shower for an entire week until the boys had to do the same amount of dishes as the girls. Our hair would get greasy. We would get smelly. We would get as gross as needed to make this change happen. Everyone would have to deal with us. The adults waved us away—oh, so cute, these girls being so adamant—until we bore down, made our case.

"Yeah," I heard my mom say, "why do the girls always have to do the dishes?"

By *girls* she meant girls *and* women because grown women refer to themselves as girls just as men refer to them as girls.

I knew my mom would eventually come through for us.

I beamed at her. Thank you.

We now understood how to use our female body to get what we wanted.

It was our first feminist protest.

Somewhere in all of this, we moved to America, to Texas. We were no longer internationals. I befriended two neighborhood girls. We swam in each other's backyard pools, zoomed our bikes through alleys. In private, I pretended to be a gorgeous woman who emerged from the ocean in a Neutrogena commercial. One afternoon, they asked if they could dye my hair blond with lemon juice.

"No," I said with crossed arms.

I had never been and would never be one to alter my physical self—and I was mad that my world thought, and therefore I thought, blond was better. They begged. They must have sniffed me out, known, as girls know about each other, that I bullied myself and so they, therefore, could do the same. We skipped into one of their bedrooms under the pretense of them showing me a new horse book. The door slammed shut. Then wham. They pushed me onto the floor. One straddled me and held my arms over my head. I flailed as the other poured lemon juice all over my hair, all over my face, until my eyes stung, stung, stung. When they flopped away from me, we were all aware a transgression had been made. I left without saying anything. On my walk through the alley back home, I cried and pulled at the dark green ivy crawling up fences, wrapped it around my arms, around and around until it tangled me up.

This was about the time my hands took over and wanted to explore beneath my underwear at night. I wouldn't let them. Nope. Not gonna do it. Gonna be good. Under my blue bedspread, they drummed on my belly, ready for something I sensed was not an okay thing to do.

Instead, my hands led me down a pool lane in the butterfly stroke. At swim practice, and during races, I beat my two legs into one tail, arced up and out of crystal-clear chlorinated water. When our coach threw his gold watch to the bottom of the pool, we hovered on the edge. What now? He spoke about the importance of breath holding, how to control the body.

"Who wants—" he began to ask, and, before he could finish his sentence, I dove, ready to return the gold up to the light.

One of my swim friends had a deathly allergy to macadamia nuts. I had never met someone with an allergy. I immediately wanted one too. What could I be allergic to? Nothing was wrong with me. I wanted something to be wrong so adults would worry over me or so I would stand out. My mother always told me my body was strong. Probably all the dirt I had eaten as a child. I fought illness off quickly. My cuts healed up with no fanfare. Nothing ever lingered in my system. No part of me was wounded.

I was out of luck.

In our American house, I would often slide an old shoebox out from our white cupboard and place it on my lap. Inside lived my mother's modeling pictures: her wearing a black hat down over one eye and pulling gum out of her red-lipped mouth, her neck arched back with mini-bicycles riding across it, her smiling face in a Japanese newspaper, a few more. These were her only copies. She had shoved them next to photo albums on a bottom shelf. I had started to take serious stock of my own beauty. I didn't want to care about beauty but somehow I did. There was something less tailored about my face. I didn't know how an unbeautiful girl could be born to a beautiful woman.

I once wanted a pair of the side-zip pants everyone else at school wore.

"They don't work on your body," my mother had said in the dressing room. The only way I knew how to deal with the sting was by getting grouchy with her. I was unable to tell her it hurt my feelings. But when my dad was out of town for work, I would sneak downstairs to sleep in her bed. She never said no. Propped up in bed with a paperback, she would slowly eat a stack of saltine crackers and butter from a paper towel with one hand and stroke my forehead with the other.

I could have stayed there forever.

One day, during my shoebox ritual, I discovered my hamster had escaped and chewed the edges of my mother's modeling pictures, destroyed them as if he had been seeking them out.

"Oh no."

Followed by a sudden and full and strange satisfaction.

For much of middle school, I made home in magnolia trees. My brothers and I biked down the street to meet up with some other boys. In their front yard, we climbed as high as possible: white flowers in spring and waxy leaves in summer. They were all boys. They were younger than me. Climbing trees, and the anticipation of climbing trees, sent a surge through me. I wanted to feel the rough bark under my palms. I wanted to do it all day long as heat pushed sweat down my nose. Move, move, move my body. When we traveled through airports as a family, I never took the escalator. I ran up the stairs two at a time. My father once suggested a dance class for me. He had loved the one he took in college. But to me then, grace and strength didn't occupy the same house. I dismissed dance as too girly and feminine.

Instead, I made myself masculine; doing so protected my sadness about beauty. I told my mom I wanted to be like the lady down the road. She had almost no breasts. "One day, you'll appreciate yours," my mother encouraged. I found sports. Longer girls could run faster than me now. I had the piss and vinegar for hurdles. It was a natural movement for me. I grinded my shoe into the sticky track, glared forward, and burst, soaring one leg over the hurdle as the other whipped around to find the ground and launch me, without a beat, toward the next hurdle. It felt like running from an animal. During practice and races, my coach would lean in over the track from the field and yell, "Good job, kiddo," as I came around each lap. My body moved faster with these words. This was my place. These were my blessings, these simple words.

But my hips were changing.

"My hip bones feel like they're moving," I explained to my mom.

"Don't worry about it, Molly," she said, and ended the conversation. My friends didn't know what I was talking about either.

I couldn't climb trees in exactly the same way.

I couldn't move the same way.

I couldn't accept the new breast buds on my chest, so I engineered a complex game of telephone to avoid feeling embarrassed in front of my mother. I asked a flat-chested friend to ask her mother to suggest to my mother that we all go on a bra-shopping expedition. But I would have rather been lying in a meadow of wildflowers and wondering about all the ways a girl could be a girl and a woman could be a woman.

The brown spots in my underwear caught my attention. Had I pooped? No. Maybe this was that period thing, but I knew almost nothing about it. Wasn't it supposed to be red?

A few days later, I wore a red skirt to our end-of-the-year school assembly.

I bled all over the seat. No. No. This couldn't be happening. Then the principal called me up to the podium to receive the Citizenship Award for being the kindest student in the school. No, no way, not now. Years of shame flushed through my small body, red from toes to forehead. Everyone, all five hundred people or so, turned to stare and smile at me for all my goodness, and the pewter silence of it almost killed me. I willed myself to slip the event program over the blood smear on the chair and walk myself on up there.

Public Announcement: Someone has entered her womanhood. Let it be known.

Despite the wet blood between my legs, no one said anything to me. I don't know who noticed and who didn't.

My mother gave me maxi pads and told me about the hook pads she had once worn as a girl. Months later, I asked her about tampons. I hated the feeling of a pad between my legs and always seemed to bleed through them in school, onto my shorts, on the car seat of our carpool driver. Like a fugitive, I stole away to the bathroom with my tampon box and read the instructions cover to cover. I was supposed to stick something the width of an entire pencil inside me.

How would it not injure me?

"Mommmm," I called, and upstairs she came.

I wouldn't let her watch. She coached me through the door. Deep breath. Go. The tampon eventually fit nice and snug. I glanced in the mirror and bust through the door. Without saying a word to my mom, I ran down the stairs and cartwheeled around the yard. Summer. Birdsong. Breeze.

I could move again.

This change granted me a station above my brothers.

Now that my period had arrived, I sighed at their ignorance. They didn't "get" anything at all. They were mere boys and I was a woman. One day, when my mother and brothers went into the mall, I waited in our Jeep with the windows down to let a hot muggy air blow through. In the backseat, I raised my legs up to stare at them: freckles, tan, slender, and they pleased me, especially because my mother had compared her legs to mine earlier that day, noting how mine were such a nicer color. Apparently, mine didn't have any veins like hers. Despite my comment at the pyramids, my mother's legs had never seemed ugly to me before. Why didn't she like her legs?

It was the last moment I would gaze upon my legs with such admiration.

Even though my mother had put a hand on my shoulder and acted like something grand had begun for me, I still considered my period a nuisance. But only because that's how everyone talked about it, that's what we were supposed to feel about it. Oh, I'm on my period. Oh, my cramps. Oh, it's such a pain. It was cool to be put out by the whole drama. Secretly, the rhythm of it had won me over, though I couldn't articulate it and I didn't understand what becoming a cycling woman meant, beyond blood and pregnancy.

I had a new body now.

But if someone had told me that blood and pee came out of two separate holes, I would have been shocked.

I knew so little of what this new body could do.

I knew so little of my femaleness.

Release

Anatomy matters to me. I want my daughter to know that hers matters, especially because our culture pretends female anatomy doesn't. We don't name it, other than with pet names. We don't discuss it. We don't educate about it. We only control it and tell it what it can't and can do. This I cannot accept. One afternoon, as I change Eula's diaper on the cabin floor, my mother gasps.

"What's that?" she says. "Looks like blisters."

"*Mom*, you've changed her diaper a thousand times. Those are her inner labia."

"Oh."

"I mean, did I not have labia as a baby?" I tease and try to keep it light.

"Of course you did, I just . . ."

I don't want to bully my mother. I had so many body questions as a girl. My mother was a different mother when I was young. She only had cloaked answers then because she herself had been given cloaked answers.

So I learned to stop asking, to shut that valve.

I'm trying to be more open with her.

She is trying too.

Sometimes it's a disaster.

Sometimes it works.

~

My mom suggests we get out. Winter has set in at twenty below. It's a choice. Emerge from the den or become cemented down. I've made efforts to go to River Road before, alone: strapped Eula to my chest and held Bru on a leash he isn't used to. But ten minutes into walking on this sunny dirt road, the warmest spot closest to us, my girl's nose would turn into a cherry and my jeans would be urine wet and the expedition would be over. What I really want to do is venture out for a long afternoon of cross-country skiing, my most cherished snow adventure. But the pressure of Eula's backpack on my bladder has made that an impossibility—at least in my current reality.

I'm seasoned now.

I squeeze the stroller into my tiny car.

We arrive and the young male cows at a farm come to the fence to greet us.

"Hey, boys," I say, as we crunch past them over ice, moving along the wide river, and eventually to a stone house. We wrap our coats tighter and my hand touches Eula's nose. She's okay. We are okay.

"This road connects all the way to Gateway," I explain when we return to the car.

"It does?" my mom says from beneath the blue scarf covering her entire face. She is so willing, so up for anything all the time. Last week, at the hot springs, Eula sucked ninety-eight-degree water up her nose and we dashed back to the changing room. So. Much. For. That. As I dressed my overheated, screaming daughter, my mother, whose hair was matted wet to forehead, somehow dressed me as she held a scrunched-up sock ready for my foot. The taking care is passed on but never leaves the source.

"Yeah," I say, "it can be muddy this time of year, but there hasn't been much snowmelt, so we should be fine. Let's do it."

"Okay, you drive, though," she says.

My tiny car has killer snow tires but almost no clearance.

We putt-putt down the narrowing road, past farmhouses, until there are no more farmhouses, and we start to slide in mud ice here and there, but I avoid the ruts. I am finally introducing my mother to something in this valley. She is no longer escorting me. I am escorting her. We slip more. I straighten the wheels and start to think about what would happen if we do get stuck, how no one knows where we are and cell phones only work in pockets out here and it's below zero and my infant daughter is with us. It gets tense, but my mom laughs with the tension and her laughter relaxes me and we move through the mud ice as people move through cycles of hope and despair, and we do not deflate. When Eula cries, I turn up the volume to Neko Case wailing about crows and love, and something about the sound and the movement and the cold and being in a car with her mama and her Mare calms her down. At a stand of shivering cottonwood trees, we come around the last bend and it feels like flying. Like we've made it through something.

~

Some people say you can make a change overnight. I am an advocate of small releases and how they eventually integrate into a sustainable change. I do my pelvic exercises. Some days. They still don't feel like a simple physical therapy. I have to unearth my entire history and make peace with every man in the world and every woman and myself in order to fully heal. Tall order. Maybe this belief is my own limitation. The more I learn about my body mechanics, the more overwhelmed I become. The pelvic bowl is, of course, connected to the whole body. To heal it, I need to also strengthen my core muscles and foot arches while stretching my hamstrings and quads and calves into a new flexibility. It requires a full-body change. It's a lot. Meanwhile, my thyroid is managed with a T3/T4 pill, a careful combination ground down at a pharmacy, so I can get through the day without a shroud wrapped around myself. Holcomb says we have to test it every three months or so and see how it goes. What is the endgame? We want to avoid an autoimmune disease. When the thyroid is off, something else is usually off, letting the person know to pay attention, please. It will help, she says, to get sleep and also foster connection.

Connection with Chris continues to be hard.

My fuse has become shorter.

My recovery time is longer. It used to take me a few hours to pull myself back together from an argument with him. Now, a week passes. I try not to think about whether this is the new permanent me or not. We haven't had a pause; we are still in the thick of something.

Later, I will name it The Dark Night of The Couple. We hash it out in the bathroom one evening. I am lying in an empty bathtub that smells of lavender, and my socks are damp from leftover shower water. He sits against the toilet. The air hangs thick with the unsaid, the almost said, the already said. If someone lit a match, we would all explode. We are trapped there for days, weeks, years. We cannot escape. I refuse to let him slip out the door, even as the ceiling crushes us. Fear rests on my lap and leans against my chest. There are grievances. There is resentment. We are a record on replay.

"I just need you to say, out loud, that you see my pain," I say.

"We cannot have this conversation out of the context of our deeper conflict," he responds. "That's really important."

"You sound like a robot."

"Someone has to be rational and un-triggered."

"You don't sound un-triggered."

"I'm trying to identify our patterns," he says.

"I appreciate that, but it would help me if you could honor me somehow. I feel like you refuse, on purpose, to see me. That disconnection is the worst."

He sighs.

"Do you want me to build our house so you can have a stable place to live, or do you want me to spend time honoring you?"

I start to cry.

His blank stare is the hardest part for me.

I'm on the edge of a cliff. I hang on, about to fall into a canyon of bitterness toward him and all men. The canyon is not of my own making. Many women have fallen into it before. My women have fallen into it before. I never wanted to be one of those women. I never wanted to detest my husband. I thought our love would keep us safe.

Somehow we sleep. In my dream, I ask a young woman how she got across the ocean and lakes and rivers and canyons and fields.

"I flew," she says.

"Oh, flying," I say.

"Like this," she explains, and leans out until her body takes flight.

~

What I learn: We rarely feel safe to fall apart. We hold it together. Then, when hardship descends and the planets and people around you happen to have aligned a certain way, a door opens. All wounds are relational wounds. The only reason I can collapse is because, despite my incontinence, my basic needs *are* taken care of—food, shelter, water, and safety. My anger is a luxury. I'm okay with this. It feels like a duty. My mother and grandmother and great-grandmother and beyond couldn't afford to scream out, not as young women. They would have lost husbands and security and who knows what else. I would rather live life with a companion. But my education and era has given me the opportunity to thrive alone if need be or if chosen. My fellow women also speak out. It is no longer so taboo. Most of us won't be burned at the stake, at least in the West. Those sisters who are still stoned or beaten or murdered elsewhere and here, they are the ones we must scream out for, speaking words they want to but cannot. When I stare out at the valley, it becomes a bowl made by the upsweep of mountains on all sides. My/our pelvic bowl is this bowl. *I can pull it up.* No one, no event, no broken moment can destroy it.

My anger is a luxury.

My anger is a luxury.

My anger is a necessity.

Recently though I wonder whether I have become attached to my anger. Devoted to it. What happens if I don't shout it out? Would I lose anything?

~

In the gynecologist's waiting room, I fiddle with my bag. We don't have a relationship. This is my yearly exam. I'm sure she's going to tell me I'm doomed. I've heard myself tell people my thyroid is fucked, my pelvic floor is fucked, and probably my hormones are fucked too. Then I apologize for my language. I've wanted to say *fuck* five thousand times until someone hears my pain. I recognize my victim mentality and also that I haven't been able to pull myself out.

When she walks into the room, her voice sounds kind.

"I know this might sound strange," I say in my blue drape. "But I need to feel something positive about my prolapse and incontinence. For better or worse, I'm sensitive and really absorb what medical professionals tell me. I know my response is my responsibility but just wanted to tell you that. I don't need you to sugarcoat, but . . ."

"Let's take a look," she says, and inserts the cold speculum.

"This looks great," she says. "You just look like a woman who's had a baby. The cystocele isn't bad. Not bad at all for pushing for five hours."

"Really?"

"Yes. You just need to be mindful of heavy lifting."

"What about the incontinence?"

"It may never be perfect, but your exercises will help."

I put the *may never be perfect* part on a wooden shelf somewhere away from my heart and focus on the fact that my vulva just looks like a woman who's had a baby. Her words aren't all that different than what the nurse told me.

"Thank you, thank you so much," I gush. "You are the kindest MD I've ever met." I want her to know she has made a difference for me.

"Oh, that means a lot. Thank you."

I hop into my clothes and skip out of there. It has become normal to me to look for a problem with my body. Maybe I've done so ever since puberty, that girl looking for a reason to be different. Maybe that has been the most dangerous act of my life. As my car eases back home, past black cows hunkered together, past snow and snow and snow, a statement appears and sifts down over me: *I am healthy. I am healthy. I am healthy.*

It is new.

What do I do with it?

I want to be aware of my body but not obsessed. I want to pass to Eula some combination of my mother's ability to roll with the punches and my ability to dig deep for truth. The middle road.

~

Eula has her first fever on the first full moon of the year. In the darkness, I hold her naked body against my chest all night long. She tosses and tosses. Hot, dry hot. Nothing soothes her. Not even my breast. I hum to her and am calm. I am always calm when someone else is ill, when someone else needs me.

The next morning, my mother comes in.

"How are you?" she asks. "First fever is always hard."

"I'm actually fine," I say, with a smile, "I didn't sleep at all, but I'm just fine."

A few days later, late at night, I go to my mom's house to chat at normal volume on the phone with a friend. When I come back to the guesthouse, nothing is as it should be. Everyone should be asleep, but Chris is holding a crying Eula in the light of the bathroom. He's inspecting her head.

"What happened?" I ask, moving toward her fast.

"She woke up screaming," he says. "I found blood on her sheets."

"What?"

We can't find any blood on her, though.

We tuck her into bed with us and assume a new tooth broke the surface.

The next morning, I scrub the small blood patch from her sheets under cold water. It is the first time I've seen her blood, my daughter's blood, the blood of our ancestors made into hers. Of course, it won't be the last time, but I don't want it to wash down the drain into the ground. Photograph it somehow. Preserve it forever.

Instead, I raise it to my lips.

~

Meanwhile, Chris continues to build our house. It is the easy but not so easy conversation between us. We were supposed to be out of the guesthouse two months ago. My parents aren't putting pressure on, but we feel the pressure. Most days, his face goes blank around anyone but Eula. He lifts her up, smooches her ears, face, hands. We show up for her even when we can't show up for ourselves, or each other. I have made the choice to be as hands-off as possible. I cannot make any emotional requests of him. I cannot say much at all. It's too much for him to hold. This detachment is unlike me, so my execution of it is sloppy.

His hands have started to go numb at night.

He can sleep only on his back.

"We should probably look for a rental," I say one evening in bed.

"We can't spend money on a rental."

"I know, but we also can't stay here much longer. It just isn't fair to my parents." My mind leapfrogs through all the people I know in town, who do we know, who has a place, how can this work, I can make this work, we can do this.

He rolls onto his stomach.

"You know what," I add, "I don't want you to worry about it. *You* are building our house. I can be in charge of figuring out where we are going to live in the meantime. I can do that, okay? That'll make it easier. Good old division of labor."

He says nothing.

Quiet as a green hill.

I must allow him his silence. In this moment, I have become someone noble, a real adult who is going to deal and isn't, for once, triggered by her husband's non-response. That's when his back starts to heave and heave and heave and heave and heave and then the sounds of his sadness emerge. My chest starts to implode—a man in tears is the underbelly, the unexpressed, the push back to a world that expects a certain definition of manhood. They say boys stop crying publicly around age seven. I've seen him cry before, often, stood on porches to say goodbye, held each other under the rain, but not recently. This is new. This is a wail, his own sort of depression, his own sort of giving up. I don't know what he needs me to be right now. If I am part of the cause, then is it okay for me to be the comforter?

I have been such forest fire for him.

I scoot closer, put my hand on his heaving back, and rub him.

I don't ask.

I know not to ask.

I know not to analyze.

~

When Eula turns nine months old, she spits peas out to see how far they can fly. I chase her crawling. She laughs hard. She bangs her wooden spoon and rejects books she's seen too much. Textiles send her eyes into another world I don't know about. She starts to fold cloth—any cloth, napkins, dish towels, rags. She is content. I've created rhythm and ritual for her. I can be proud of that.

There is one photo from my labor.

I've never seen it.

Chris shows me.

I am in transition, my cervix opening from eight to ten centimeters, arms flung over the tub, the messy bun of my brown hair, about to start pushing, probably fifteen minutes away from going to the hospital though we didn't know it. I see that hopeful calm woman and want to bring her into my arms. Maybe she needs to pull me into her arms—remind me of how to labor, how to be separate from fear. She has a message for me. *It's time to move forward.* Here again. I've developed a true compassion for those who rage and make poor decisions. Beneath that swell of anger is some form of pain, and beneath that, divinity. I've touched it a few times at the lowest of the low. *No matter, you are here now.*

Dear women.

I write an email to my closest friends to ask them to help me mark this moment. I make a conscious choice to take a turn in the road.

We can be good.

We can set intention.

There are so many moments when we think we've changed. There are so many moments when I think I've changed. These are not false, but they are not static either. How many times in my life have I decided I would will myself to be fine now and forever? The expression *nine months in, nine months out* refers to what exactly? Someone once told me baby steps. This is one of those.

~

Alternative medicine and bodywork can become a wormhole for me. I don't require scientific studies to prove it works. I want to try it all because every experience leads me closer to my body, myself, the natural world around me, leaves, trees. It's an option many of us don't realize we have, or can't afford to have. Other than naturopathy with Holcomb, I haven't allowed myself to open that door recently: acupuncture, massage, or singing bowls played over my body. I keep investigating and investigating and it's time to focus on the one resource I always have.

Myself.

Unless I can trade with someone; in this instance, her services for my writing coaching. I scrape ice off my windshield and drive to town to get a Mayan abdominal massage. It's a technique to heal and realign the uterus. My uterus seems okay, but I want to be in touch with my pelvis and all its contents. Dark room, incense, oils, deep sound of the woman's voice, and her confident, strong touch. She rubs my belly in circles and then strokes inward from two parts of the pelvis and then two parts of the ribs. Then she asks me to do it, to massage myself and go through the process.

I begin.

"Wait," she stops me. "Breathe and pull yourself from head to root."

I do and it feels like descending in an elevator.

Down.

Down.

Down.

I've tried to embody this way many times but have never gotten there and suddenly I'm there and stunned. There is my uterus. Hi. I've rubbed around my belly only a few times. The woman asks me to send my uterus love for growing my baby and bleeding for me. Yes, okay, I understand. But this sort of self-care is hard for me, why is this hard for me? I'm here. I can't let myself take myself seriously. I start to feel bad for my uterus, poor thing, not getting the love from me she deserves. Then my history with self-hate hits me. Tears don't bother to form slowly. They catapult out from my face, and my lips tremble, a tremble that moves across the canvas of my throat down to my chest. She notices me try to will it away and continue my self-massage, but my hands cannot move.

She puts her hands on me.

"There, there, no need to go anywhere else, just place your hands there and send love."

~

Afterward, for days, I lie awake at night with my hands on my uterus. I don't hear much—only a dark warm silence, restful even. I don't have acres of patience. I want contact. Actual words. Made from the alphabet. Instead, images come: palm trees and paper reams and wooden shoes and tigers and mossy rocks and, of all things, a spatula.

There is a wilderness in my uterus.

My cognitive self cannot function there. My uterus does not theorize about what she is or isn't because an organ operates on felt-sense, responds that way, acts upon that way, shifts that way. How is it that she has known to bleed every twenty-eight days? How did she grow and give shelter to a baby? How did she know when, the precise moment, to start contracting around that baby? As the days pass, my body and I finally enter an honest conversation. It has received many instructions and accusations from me. It seems confused about this. There is a zigzag feeling. That's how I know what it says. We *are* on the same team, I assure it.

I won't ever betray you. Even when I do.

~

My car moves down the snowy road at dawn. I arrive with other hot-spring pilgrims and, under fluorescent lights, swim laps near a

woman who lowers herself from a wheelchair into the pool. It's remarkable how people make peace with what is. My legs flutter and
take me deep and up and somersaulted. Here, only here, do I remember how capable my body is of graceful and athletic movement. When
you know incontinence doesn't matter because you are in water, the
body does not constrict. There is no holding.

I've come to appreciate simple acts of my past—stepping into a
hot shower and controlling the urge to pee, laughing so hard with
friends everyone has to cross legs because you're all "going to pee"
even though you're not, spotting a large rock and running fast to leap
over it and then land beyond like a cat.

My goggles fog up. I rinse them as another woman enters the hot
water fully clothed. A few older men emerge from the cold plunge
like seals, or gods. I make my way to the silent outdoor pool where
darkness has begun to peel away from the sky. Tread water. Stare up
at fir trees. A Tom Waits song enters me. Then words, not his, but
my words matched to his rhythm, a song for Eula: I put limes on the
table and string flowers from the bed, when it rains hard tomorrow,
we'll listen to the drum overhead. Other lines about my arms always
open for her, about how we'll dance wild in the spring of April. I can't
stop. Then the line I've needed arrives.

I've got a body full of stars.
I've always had them.
I've forgotten them.

Afterward, in the parking lot, I face my car toward a trailer park
and start to tap on my chest. The science of tapping yourself into
health seems legit. I don't know why we all aren't doing it all the
time, or why I've only just begun and probably won't continue with
any regularity. For now, I am the lady bundled up in a down jacket
and hat who taps on her forehead, her wrist, her clavicle, her heart,
her eyebrows.

What is that lady doing? the people walking out wonder.
She is caught between trying everything and nothing all at once.

~

In the grocery store, people continue to tell me that Eula is a serious baby.

"Yep, she *is* a studious one," I hear myself respond. "But she smiles at home."

Lauren tells me to say to people, "She just doesn't like you." Why the hell am I apologizing for my daughter, for the exquisite intensity of my daughter, for her no-bullshit detector? People prefer girls who smile at first glance. It scares them to have a girl look right into their eyes.

I told my mother the other day that I'm intentional, not intense.

Not intense the way people define *intense*.

"Yes," she said, "I see that."

Thank you. After years of being called intense by my family. I would like to change my tendency to be a bulldozer determined to rearrange the earth. That aggression doesn't serve anyone. But when did intense become a bad thing to be? Intense is laser eyes, clear mind, focused, articulate tongue. It isn't bad for a man. Our culture believes an intense woman is a catastrophe. I'm tired of the inevitability of this paradigm.

~

After a long day of teaching, I push the door open into my mom's cabin. She has tied twine to a plastic laundry basket and is pulling Eula around in this boat. Wooden spoon in hand, Eula grunts when my mom stops, grunts again to say *More*. I wouldn't have thought of this simple game.

It's been six months since I returned to work—meeting with clients about their projects and teaching four classes a semester. No one would guess I struggle. I crack jokes about the hardship of early motherhood or sleep deprivation. I'm not trying to hide it. But everyone thinks I'm normal. One of my students tells me she sees clarity in my eyes, no pain, no subterfuge. Who is that woman she is talking about? Where is she? I squeeze my professional life into two full days with a lot of catch-up in the evenings. My mother watches Eula one day a week—they make construction-paper art projects and look through all her jewelry. Chris watches her the other day, takes her skiing around the field or to Home Depot to talk to Gary the plumber. During my four solo days with my daughter, we make meals and do laundry.

I know there is value in her watching daily tasks.

I know there is value in not entertaining her.

We also sing.

I'm trying to keep myself steady.

I stay steady until something with Chris turns sour again. Here's the honest consideration: let's say my subconscious, or even conscious, self was preventing me from healing in order to both get Chris's attention and punish him. It's likely. It's ugly. I haven't allowed myself to voice my continued concern that I cannot heal my body while living in the climate of this marriage. All I want him to do is recognize what I've undergone. He did, sort of, the other day. We sank into the car together (my request and my asking my mom to take Eula). Our taxed breath fogged up the windows. His gray wool jacket was covered in sawdust from work. This would be our culminating moment after almost two years, since my pregnancy, of me continually asking him to verbally honor me—and him not doing so. He read off the list I wrote and gave to him: *I honor you for carrying our daughter for almost ten months, I honor you for vomiting that entire time, I honor how difficult it must feel to pee on yourself daily, I honor . . .* He was kind. I cried until my nose was raw because his body language indicated that his words were only out of duty. He was following orders he thought "good" husbands should follow. When he said, "Let's do this every night," with a distant voice, something in me broke again. Were we playing pretend? Were we in some film where I played the wife? I wanted him to come up with his own words. I wanted him to care enough to plan and organize and initiate the whole thing. As if he were the keeper of a magic potion that would allow me to heal. When the car door shut, I didn't know where or who I was. My vow to turn a corner had turned into a brick wall.

"That's so simple and great," I say to my mom when she looks up.

"You kids used to love your cardboard-box boats," she says.

I scoop Eula up and nuzzle her to my face.

"How's Chris feeling?" my mom asks.

The question launches me into a rant about how men can't deal, how Chris has a cold and he can't function, like he can't form a sentence it is so painful, and I want to scream, "Oh please. Are you joking? It's that bad? Try feeling like shit, so much worse than you've ever felt for nine, no, ten months straight, and then going through childbirth, and then feeling even worse, a thyroid that doesn't work, hormones probably askew, loss of continence and therefore loss of a basic human dignity, with almost zero sleep and a child dependent on your breast, your mood, your everything, but you show up and smile and sing and create rhythm for her despite it all. Try that. A cold. Whatever. Mothers are the only ones capable of never getting a break. I wake up with Eula at five forty-five, whether I'm sick or not, when you can't muster the energy, because you aren't a morning person."

I'm aware of the superlatives flying out my mouth.

"I know," she says.

"I'm losing faith in men," I sigh. "And I have one of the best."

"You really do," she agrees.

I don't want to become that bitching woman. I really don't. Though, if a friend ranted and released in the same way, I would hold the space for her, wouldn't let her define herself as a bitching woman. I've never hated men. I don't want to believe they are less resilient. I don't know whether I'm mad at Chris or all men or the unchecked masculine in our world and in all of us. My cells are in a holding pattern about it. As I watch my mom pulling Eula around in her laundry basket, the strength of women moves like a tidal wave over me. I want to chest bump every woman on the planet.

~

At the end of February, we move out of the guesthouse. It is time. My parents need it as a rental, and we want to respect that. Our friend Rebecca has invited us to live in her basement in town for free and we have offered to pay some rent, something for utilities, something. We'll keep her and her infant son company while her husband works out of town.

The car is packed.

Two backpacks full of clothes, a crib, and my Costco-size box of *Always* Extra-Long Pads with Wings. Rebecca said it's okay for us to bring Bru but he's too big and he would probably dog-hair their entire home. He'll stay with my parents until we move into our house, sometime late this summer.

"Come here, sweets," I say, and I gather Eula, who is nearly one year old and crawls like a gorilla now, with one fist, one flat hand. We walk around the concrete floor of the guesthouse. Say goodbye to the fan, fireplace, and Mexican giraffe. I remind her that we labored here together and she grew almost her first full year here. Part of me grieves and settles into nostalgia. The other part is depending on the energy of a geographic switch.

"This is the last time we'll be here as we have been," I say, and she cocks her head at me and starts to whimper. I tell her it's okay, but somehow she understands we are leaving. She waves goodbye to the trees without a prompt from me.

Goodbye, trees.

My mom stands by our car wearing her father's old wool hat and her standby black stretch pants. She knows how to move across oceans with infants. This move is nothing.

Goodbye, Mom.

Goodbye, Mare.

Thank you.

We will be back. But in our own house—nearby, but separate.

On our drive over, I know we'll see my mother in a few days, so easy. In moments like these I always reference the story of my orphaned Irish great-great-grandmother who, as a twelve-year-old, stepped onto a ship bound for America with her two siblings and never returned home.

We are all descended from the remarkable.

In the backseat, Eula laughs at her book.

Her hee-haw laugh is my laugh.

When we arrive, the shift to town is noticeable. Gone is most of the wild. Gone are the owls. Gone are the cranes and mountain lions, the presence of a creek, the open, the trees holding us up with their roots. The weather isn't gone, though. Chris unloads our duffel bags, and I help where I can. With Eula on one hip and small bags in the other hand, it occurs to me that my incontinence has made literal movement through life difficult. Sleep deprivation is a heavy smothering blanket, but maybe it wouldn't have knocked me down so hard if we had had our own home, or if I could walk to the car or out of a grocery store without feeling like my organs were going to fall out of my vagina. Maybe I could have been a normal sleepy mother. Is there such a thing? I've never been scared of effort. But this kind of effort has no name. It has shorted me out.

I try to be kind to myself.

After dinner, I take Eula downstairs for bed. I explain this will be our home for a while, and we go about making it so. We say good night to the music speaker, trees outside the window, wooden boxes, zebra, map, and the lights. We will do this same bed ritual for months.

Over the next week, Rebecca unloads what she has been holding. She, unlike me, has been alone. She tells me how she has lost her inherent confidence since becoming a mother. She was so in her skin as an adolescent. I listen and notice grief catch in my throat—grief for her, grief for me, for having missed that *in my skin* knowing that could have been when I was that age. We pause. We feed the babes some salmon and egg yolk and sauerkraut and zucchini. We remember to eat some ourselves too even though we would rather eat bread and butter.

The conversation continues, in the minutes that make up each day.

This, we decide, is how living should be.

The village. No nuclear-family-in-one-house mumbo jumbo. And yet we all do it.

We take the babes to our local museum to check out geckos. It's our ploy to get out of the house in winter. After two laps, my pad is soaked and I tell Rebecca I won't be able to carry Eula up the stairs to the kid floor without wetting my pants completely. She grabs Eula, and up we go. I follow and watch Rebecca's strong biceps as she hips both babes on her slender frame. Neither of us knows that in less than a year her Lyme disease will flare. She'll be in a prison of seizures, and body breakdown will, eventually, surface. No matter what a woman seems to be there is always a layer beneath. Why are so many of our bodies suffering? For now, she appears to be the goddess mother I can't be. The numbness starts in my chest and moves out to my limbs. Just feel the sadness, don't numb. But numb is how I've learned to self-protect.

~

She's been at it for an hour in the shadowy dark. It's well past her bedtime, but I won't pry her away. Her ten-month-old body is working something out. Her front teeth have started to come in. She leans against the carpeted stairs in this new home. It's her first encounter with climbing to another level. Lifts one leg, looks down, picks up a foot, as if willing it to do something. Next she arcs her back, reaches up into nothingness and talks about it, moan, groan, chirp, dadadada-dadadada. I let it happen because what else can I do? There is so much golden hope in this moment. She becomes a bear cub. She becomes, perhaps for the first time, completely unaware of where her mama is. Then, with a bolt, she crawls up one step, pauses for an instant, realizes what has happened, then slides back down, retreats back to safe space. And this, yes, is how it works for all of us, I think, sitting there, my back against the wall, watching my daughter find ascension.

~

What I learn: No part of the body is isolated. The pelvic bowl and feet mirror one another. Fallen arches can indicate weak bowl. My flat feet may be part of the equation. From the beginning of this journey, I've sensed pronounced collapse on the right side of my pelvic bowl, much like my more collapsed right arch. Strengthen the foot and see what happens. Same story with the jaw. Midwives know to tell a laboring woman to loosen her mouth—no clench. When you release the jaw, the cervix can ideally dilate as it needs to. I remember that sensation. Our mouth is connected to our root is connected to our feet. It all operates as a movement. A prolapse can often be a result of misaligned posture. Women know, instinctively, how to walk with a curve in our body. It's a biological benefit. But how many hours have I sat in a chair—in school, at college, at jobs, as a writer, right now? Humans were never meant to sit. I have also wanted to hide my body. Don't poke my butt out. Don't sway. There is an unlearning that must happen. Untuck my tail. Invite myself back into movement.

~

We go to visit friends and family on the East Coast. On the airplane, Chris and I snuggle our faces together as Eula stands on us, ooos and ahhhs at everyone. She's a croaker these days, sounds like a pterodactyl orating to the masses. People will ask me, "What's she like?" Studious. Shy. Silly. Observer. I can name these qualities, and they are true, but I want to practice saying, "That might change." That being shy or silly or any category isn't for life, if *she* doesn't want it for life. I want to notice her in a way that she notices me noticing.

In New York, one of my close friends does a bodywork session on me. She tells me I've always had a deep reservoir but don't have access to it now because I'm blocked. My diaphragm is crammed up in my chest. Emotions have no way to process and can't reach my organs.

It feels to her like my body is cut in half.

"I don't know how to do this healing and do everything else," I say.

"You will do it," she says. "Just be gentle with yourself."

In the early morning, as we stare out at a blue-dawn city, Eula, who thought the skyscrapers were trees, bites the hell out of my elbow flesh. I make a silent deal with her. If this buys me another hour, another fifteen minutes of sleep, bite away, I'll take it.

The movement.

At night, she won't wind down.

"We were here together once," I tell her, "when you were in Mama's belly." I sat nauseous on this bed, read about baby sign language, and finally connected with tears to the fetus within me. Now we sign every day—please, more, all done, milk. She nods and spin spin spins, scoots herself safely off the bed, reaches for everything, does side somersaults, waves at the elephant mobile, cackles, arches her back and then, when she finds my hairbrush, we are all hairbrush for an hour. I show her that it brushes my hair. She tries it on her own hair, slow at first and then swats at my head, trying to help me brush. I see practice as integral to life now. She is on the verge of walking and must use all her muscles to get there. I am on the verge of healing and must use all my muscles to get there. This back-and-forth goes on forever, in the dark, with the sounds of sirens and human bustle below. I love this moment of teaching her how to groom herself, all that is implicated, all the beauty and obligation and expectation of woman with her hair. None of that is here. The brush is a tool. I am her mother and she is my daughter and we can delight in this act, just like my mother showed me with her Mason Pearson hairbrush.

Because we are on vacation and away from our storm, Chris talks openly to our dear friends. In the corners of apartments, I sit and listen. He is not talking to me directly, even though he is. He thinks birth *is* more traumatic for the partner than the woman. "How?" someone asks. Then, without drama, he shares that my eyes were closed the whole time and I didn't see the monitor with our child's dangerously low heartbeat, or the nurses from the OR ready to wheel me away, or the stress on everyone's faces, or the look on my own face. I was an animal in a flood of hormones. He wasn't. He lived it. I see his point. I see the best supporting masculine wanting credit. I want to interrupt and say that he's never given birth, for one, and suffering isn't a contest, but then I'd have to live up to that truth myself. For days, I think about what he has said, how it might extend to everything we've lived. Maybe it's more of a heartbreak to watch someone deteriorate than be the one who deteriorates. Maybe it's worse to witness an unraveling than to unravel. I've always told him I'd rather be the one dead in an avalanche than the one who loses him to an avalanche.

Where do we meet then?

How do we meet each other again?

We take the subway and head over to Riverside Park with Eula. She cranes her head out the stroller, stares at each person, at each dog, each tree. She would kiss them all if she could. This will be the first time Chris and I have shown her a place we knew before her.

"We lived here six years ago," I say out loud.

I used to jump rope here to train my muscles. We used to roller-blade together and laugh as we hopped curbs and corners. We would eat a baguette and avocado and watch the sunset over the Hudson. Chris used to find trees that meant something to him and then take my hand to show me, the bark, the leaves, the height as he wrapped his arms around my waist.

These are the moments I want to share with her.

These are the moments I want to remember with him.

This moment could be us, the new family, lying on a picnic blanket, intertwining our legs, and marveling at the trees, at each other, at bringing our daughter, our healthy co-creation, here. But I can't get on the ground because my pad is overflowing and I didn't bring another. I used to say "I'm peeing on myself" to Chris but he no longer acknowledges that I'm even speaking when I say it. His silence in response to my plea has become a pain so constricting I cannot go there. I want to be joyful for my loved ones so I continue to smile and comment on the spring smell of trees. I don't tell him how hard it is for me to be in the place my body once moved and jumped and played. I don't tell him how my pelvic floor feels extended after the long walk on concrete. I don't tell him how much I miss him, us. I don't tell him about the metal wrecking ball sitting on my chest, how the grief is so heavy I can't squirrel out from under it. I don't tell him any of this because he's heard it before and it's all mine.

I try to be someone good.

I open the packet of raspberries we just bought.

I feed one to Eula and one to Chris and one to myself until we are feeding each other and covered in stains. Forget about who you thought you would be in this moment. Just forget about it. Move on. When the wrecking ball squeezes the breath out of me again, my hand comes to my chest and rubs. I get up and tell them I just want to see that tree over there and I walk to it and lean against it in a way that won't appear to others like sadness and beg it to help me keep it together. Just for now. Please. I cannot drag my family into more grief.

~

We fly home and then across the country to San Francisco—our travel for the year lumped into two weeks. Chris stays home to work, so we make it a female trip. My mom and I push the stroller up a sidewalk near my friend's home. The air is gray and not all that warm and smells of flowers.

"Look at those bottlebrush," she says, pointing to a tree with red fuzzy caterpillar-like flowers all over it.

"Hmmm," I nod.

"They remind me of you," she offers.

"They *do*. Why?"

"The streets of Sydney were covered in them when I was pregnant with you. I used to walk to the market. I walked everywhere. Remember that brass gong? I bought it the day I found out I was pregnant with you."

"Really? I never knew that."

"I did," she says, and smiles.

"That's so something I would have done," I say. As we continue, I'm struck by my younger mother's purchase, how she made a symbol out of a moment, how I didn't know that she did that. Of course she does.

It's a short trip. On our way to the airport, I ask my friend's husband to carry my suitcase down the steep steps for me. I have to—or else. Is this my body now, is this who I am now? My mom is waiting on the sidewalk by her rental when we drive by. Without skipping a beat, she opens the trunk and hurls her suitcase in. My friend comments on how impressed she is that my mom didn't ask for help with something heavy, that her mom, most moms this age, would have. Not my mom. It's who she is. It's who I used to be. I want to be just like her.

~

It's the end of April. Eula is one day away from being a one-year-old. Chris has gone to buy groceries. Rebecca is out of town, so we have the house to ourselves. Right now, at 5 p.m., my water broke a year ago. Labor began. That labor represented all other labors—a passage of all the ages. I notice the time and hold Eula to my chest. We've been dancing to flamenco but now we waltz across the carpet listening to the ethereal sound of Icelandic music. The sun descends as aspens flutter beyond the window. I smell her head and a river of tears pours out of me, my whole body remembering, as if on cue, how we began this journey. "I love you, I love you," I say, as we dance and dance and spin, but there is no way to express such gratitude. Eula sees a dog run by outside and kicks her legs out. I put my turtle mouth to her turtle mouth and we smile at each other with our eyes.

That night, Chris and I make a dinner of pasta, pancetta, peas, and goat cheese. We drink white wine and huddle close. We talk about how our daughter is preparing to walk. She nurses like a hippo, all the time, standing, sitting, grabbing, laughing, and giving me the sign for milk, a squeeze of the hand, proud of herself for making the connection. He sets himself up on the floor. I've asked him to paint a sandhill crane in red on a handmade drum for her first birthday gift. He has an affinity for cranes; I call her my firebird; cranes fly overhead and croak their croak often, so much so that Eula will one day shock a city friend of ours when she points to a bird in a book and calls it "crane." While he designs and dips a brush in red, I write her a long letter that doesn't feel adequate enough because how do I explain her to herself, how do I explain anything about this first year?

I wish I had a letter like this from my mom.

I wish she had one from hers.

~

We've driven out to my parents' home and our soon-to-be home to celebrate Eula's birthday. Her dried umbilical cord rests in my pocket. I've been waiting to bury this cord and make ceremony. What a day. What a warm, brown, still day. We left our wool hats in the car. My cheeks feel warm. I greet the band of cottonwoods with a nod. They remember. While my parents bustle around in the cabin, Chris and I get ready to climb the hill with Eula.

"My whole body is buzzing," I say, and I squeeze him, squeeze Eula, and Bru.

The moment will beget other movement. I know so. I want so. Doesn't everything change after the first year, don't people start to break the surface again? That's what they tell you—the postpartum period is officially over at three months or nine months or a year, but it doesn't go beyond.

That demarcation would seem absurd to a more seasoned mother. *This* is hope.

"I love our life," I say, and smile at him.

"I'm glad, babe."

"Do you know if we have a trowel?" I ask.

"I don't know," he says, as he puts Eula into the carrier on his chest.

"We probably need one."

"Why?"

"I want to bury the cord, not leave it there to blow away."

"We can put some rocks on it," he says, and then adds, "If you want a trowel, you can find one. I'm not responsible for knowing where the trowel is."

What I hear is: Don't fret, Don't Ask for Help, Don't Make This a Big Deal.

What I feel is: Disconnection. Moment ruined.

"This matters to me," I say as the wrecking ball slams onto my chest, and my legs move fast to the guesthouse, away, and when I collapse on the bed, I cannot get up, no rising from this place I labored with Eula a year ago, at this time, where we breathed so well together. I try to breathe and remember me, the laboring woman, and trust that all will be well, but I'm not sure I can ever get up again.

This physical response comes from somewhere beyond that one moment.

Eventually, they come in, I get up, and we go on a walk.

I carry the now-found trowel.

My man and my daughter and my dog go ahead of me. I stay back. Alone. I weep along the ditch near our soon-to-be house. My body falls again, on wet ground. Maybe this is what needs to happen. He looks back at me and stops. But he has no energy to move toward me, and actually I don't want him near me anyway.

"Honor me, fucker," I scream into my hands so no one can hear.

We make it to the plateau.

Eula starts to eat snow.

"We can't do this right now," Chris says, and I know he's right but I don't want him to be right about anything. We don't do it, even though it's her actual birthday and the spring weather is all small hail and then sun and it's so damn beautiful. When we get back down from the plateau, he hugs me. The touch calms me enough, but I keep my distance. He doesn't feel like someone I know at all. We stand by the creek. I pick up sticks and hand them to Eula. She's still in his arms. I don't want to transfer my energy. She watches brown water flow by and then I look at my watch.

"There it is," I say. "You were born."

I press my lips to her forehead.

I stand apart and remember a memory I'm not even sure is true—how, after they sewed me up, they wheeled me to the new room as Chris stayed in the delivery room and held Eula in his arms skin to skin, and my parents came through the emergency room door, saw me on my way, quick hug, and continued past me to go meet their grand-daughter. How I, the vessel who had done my job, was carted away.

~

I ask Chris to come with me to my doctor visit with Holcomb. I want him to hear so he can be part of my healing process.

"Sure, babe," he agrees with no resistance. This hot and cold we exist in with each other is unlike anything pre-pregnancy. He calls it whiplash. I can see him as my destroyer one minute and then my savior the next. I dart like a snake from this to that. I can't know yet that I am finally connecting to my feminine. She, by essence, flows between emotions. But she is also skilled at it. I'm not skilled yet. I only do damage. My inconsistency has made me unsafe to him. We are emotionally unsafe to each other. Yet we've been ravenous for each other recently—on the carpet, blinds open, while runners run by at dusk, over and over again, as our daughter sleeps in the basement. We tend a tenuous connection. He has made it clear that he will not budge. He cannot honor me the way I need unless my anger toward him gets directed in healthier ways. He is right but some part of that equation still doesn't sit right with me.

We sit in her office. I want to be holding hands but we aren't.

Holcomb glances through the blood work and saliva test and tells me my hormones are out of balance: high estrogen and low progesterone. We could consider some progesterone supplement. My thyroid, however, is looking great. My body is actually doing the healing. I've moved out of the red zone for a potential autoimmune disease.

"It's still there. But it's far less acute," she explains with a smile.

"Really?"

I don't know what to do with this good news. There are other issues still and new issues, but this big one is actually healing. I didn't think healing would happen. On many levels, I've courted my wound, been seduced for years and years by the false power of sickness and sadness and anger. They have purpose, but aren't they meant to pass through, not lodge? Has my darkness and struggle made me interesting to myself and therefore interesting to others? I've never been curious about my joy. As we leave the office and walk past crocuses and the green flush of spring, I start to acknowledge the trench of my own making. Chris glides next to me and shows his relief at the good news when he takes hold of my hand.

"This is great. You *are* healing," he offers. "You've been waiting for a reason to take care of your body your entire life. You've wanted to heal and heal deeply."

"I know," I say, and rest my head on his shoulder.

At the pharmacy, the progesterone troches stack up as *another* medication to me. They give me vanilla-flavored. Okay. I will start them soon. They should help with mood and perhaps the prolapse too. Somehow, less than twenty-four hours after being told my body is healing itself, before any new medicine, a few miracles happen. I dance with Eula and don't pee on myself. My thighs feel and even look stronger. I stop wearing my pads at home because I don't want to become dependent on them. My whole body becomes a hawk to me. May as well spread my wings and fly. I tell Chris I will take on our food situation. We haven't been able to dial in our cooking of meals, between work and parenting. I have time to make Eula gorgeous food but never enough for us. I am still trying to release my fear of domesticity, of being a woman at home who cooks.

The next day, Eula feeds herself a bite of chicken. Then she feeds me. Then tucks a piece of it into the orchid's soil to feed it. Why not?

~

Someone recently told me about a friend whose pregnancy was easy, no nausea, a little tiredness, but not much, and the birth, oh, the birth, only four hours and a cinch, and the baby has already slept through the night for a week. Apparently, the new mother is really low-key, super low-key.

It must help to be low-key.

I never wanted to be a low-key woman.

Do I now?

I'm trying to hold on to this new possibility that my body, that I, am heal-able. Release my outrage down the creeks and rivers and back to the ocean. My ears are open for how—how to do so. A woman at a dinner shares a story with a group of us. On a walk, she once saw a mountain lion kill a deer. Her mother heard and put her in front of a medicine man for the next four days: part of their Navajo tradition.

"And they were telling me that it was a warning," she explained, "to stay with the goodness in me, to not choose the bitterness."

"Thank you," I tell her, "I need that. Thank you."

The next morning, I welcome spring. Beyond our tiny basement window, an aspen shakes itself awake. My legs are propped up, and Eula points to the birthmark on my hip.

"Yeah," I say, "that's my birthmark. You have one right here and here." I stroke her hairline where a noticeable dark freckle has always been and then point to two on her ankles. She crawls to the black sheets hanging around her crib and starts to drape them, an elaborate dance of folds, this child of folding, folding, folding. When she is done, she grabs a diaper from her basket and comes back to bed. She grins at me and puts it between my legs, as if she is going to put it on me.

"If only you knew, girl," I smile at her.

Then she crawls right up to my face, nose to nose, and plants a kiss on my mouth.

It's her first voluntary kiss.

~

In the outdoor pool at the hot springs, my legs wave in the water and what comes to me is this: "Thank you, fat, for protecting me all these years. I needed you, but I don't anymore. I'm ready to expose my muscle, myself." Under the cloudy sky, I hook my feet on the metal ladder and float back. Warm water flows over my body until the only part at surface is my nose.

I am in a cave, soft cave, womb, my mother's, yes, but a larger one, an everywoman sort of womb. She tells me to reshape my rage. It is to be used but used well. I've been rejecting my own divine feminine all these years—scared of her, unsure of her, mad at her. But she is always here and willing to give, and this has been my opportunity to connect.

Pat-Pat and Mare and Eula.

I get to remake my womanhood.

I see an old woman in the changing room, must be at least eighty-five years old, her skin as white and translucent as a moth wing.

"Hello," she winks at me.

"Hi," I say, and think *another teacher.* Pay attention. She is naked and wrinkled and sagging and stunning and wipes her feet off with paper towels, then oils her body slowly. Such care. I've never cared for my body that way. Part of my low-maintenance-woman persona. Chris has been asking me for years to step into the feminine goddess I want to be but don't admit to wanting to be. My mother taught me how to moisturize my face, brush my hair, wanted to teach me how to decorate myself.

Not for me, I said. Those things are empty, trivial, stupid patriarchy.

I didn't know they could be self-honoring.

I didn't know about the importance of that pleasure.
I don't want to be good.
I want to be whole.
"Gorgeous day," the woman says to me as she walks out.

~

What I learn: Women are doorways. Not doormats. I already know so but relearn it every day. Long ago, and not long ago, land-based people organized their lives around menstruation. Many evolutionary anthropologists believe that structure was instigated by women in order to protect children and provide the right food for pregnant and nursing mothers. In effect, it made sure the human race survived. Rituals began with the moon. Most indigenous cultures have a long-held belief in the Great Mother and the sanctity of menstruation. A woman's blood is considered as precious as gold.

Of course, even the most unsuspecting cultures honor the female—almost in secret, it seems, a holdover from another era. Many churches and cathedrals have an oval archway door (vulva) that leads into the dark sacred space (womb). The vulva shape repeats all over nature: an open door, a passageway out for every human, a place to transform.

Women can teach me, us, how to live inside of mystery and awe.
Doorways.

~

Mid-afternoon, I come home from work. My mom has been watching Eula at Rebecca's house. They don't hear my car. I lean against wood siding and peek through the large window to see them lying on the carpet with Eula flopped over Mare's belly, both of them laughing donkey laughs with each other. Sun beats on my back, a breeze, a bird, my heart, and I watch for a moment, lock the scene into my body, then knock. They grin at me but stay spun in their honey moment.

Grandmother.
Granddaughter.

My teachers.

Later that evening, Eula and I sit outdoors and she walks for the first time, from concrete onto grass—nine bold steps.

~

Summer has arrived. Eula waddles around in a green world. She watches the play of shadow and light. We are about to move back to the land. The house will be ready in August; in the meantime, we will live in our sweet yurt, all two hundred square feet of it. I could go on and on about how blessed I am. I start to notice how my incontinence changes with my menstrual cycle. The first two weeks, all is generally well, minus jumping or lifting. After ovulation, everything loosens and the closer my body gets to bleeding the more my bladder can't hold. This gives me one more piece to my puzzle.

"You know," my mother barks one day, "you just might have to consider surgical intervention." She knows better than to say that to me. Something must be bothering her. She must want to hurt me.

I stand in her kitchen and say nothing.

My armor starts to lock into place, slides over my chest and stomach first.

"I'm just saying, it is probably an important option," she adds as I move to behind the counter, far away from her.

"Mom, it's not helpful to hear that. Just because some people take the easy way out doesn't mean I will. I'm not that way. I've never been that way." *The easy way out* was offensive and not the right thing to say. I watch myself do what people do in arguments: pass my hurt on to her as a way to diffuse it away from me. But really doing that just magnifies it for everyone.

She starts to cry.

"I just need appreciation," she says, and holds her scrunched face. It always hurts to see my mother cry, turns me right into a soft snail.

"I do so much," she continues. "I've given you so much of myself. What's the problem? I don't understand." Everything she says is true. I don't know what it has to do with me having surgery but clearly what we say initially is often not what we mean or even want to say.

For her to say this is the start of a breakthrough for her, a shift in a caretaking role she's played her whole life with her children and others.

"I'm sorry," I whisper. "I haven't thanked you enough. I don't know why. I'm sorry." But my mind tracks back to all of the apologies and thank-yous. I want to string them up on a laundry line and count them. Have I withheld? I don't tell her that deep connection with anyone but Eula has felt like a burden to me—either rife with potential hurt or me as caretaker at a time where I have little to give. I want to offer more connection to my mother. We all start as a released egg waiting to be fertilized, hoping for the very first contact and connection of life.

There is so much to release.

There is so much for my mom to release.

There is so much of me to release.

A few days later, she comes over to Rebecca's house and we all sit on the couch together. Eula lifts my shirt and pokes my belly button. I tell her that's what connected me to Mare. Then she lifts Mare's shirt and my mom says, "Oh look." I love that she is willing to show her whole body to Eula.

"And that connected Mare to Pat-Pat," I say.

"And *this*," I coo, smooching her belly button, "is what connected you to me."

It's strange and common that humans come from humans.

Eula scampers up to me and brushes my hair out of my face.

Such gentle touch, this girl. She studies my face, points to my eyes, and smiles. Then she flops backward onto Mare.

I see you. I see you too.

And Took Note of Her Shape

The same summer I got my period was the same summer a stranger touched my vulva. My parents took us on a trip to Paris. In our small hotel room, my brothers and I took turns with my new red Kodak camera, snapping pictures of each other lounging like *artistes* on the wrought-iron balcony. We ate croissants and cringed at the smell of Camembert. I was twelve, the age when girls have stick legs and puffy lips. The foreign language thawed something within me. As we walked on paved and cobbled streets, I stole private glances at my reflection in glassy buildings. I wore my favorite pair of short white shorts and made sure to gloss my lips. Men walking on the street shot side-glances at me—real men. I didn't know how to react but the heat inside me grew. Never in my life had I been the pretty one. I did exactly seventy push-ups every morning. Seven was my favorite number. I practiced this new female power—swaying my hips, pouting my mouth, poking out my breasts.

On our way up the Eiffel Tower, we were shoved into a massive freight elevator, packed hip to hip. My mom and brothers ended up in one corner, my dad and I in another. I held his hand but people shoved between us. I kept holding on and my arm was awkwardly extended all the way out, even though we couldn't see each other. When the elevator doors closed, it went dark and stuffy and gross armpit smell. People were whispering, carrying on conversation, all squashed together. The man in front of me pressed very close—and I thought, Strange. As the elevator jostled up slowly, a hand lightly brushed the inside of my thigh. It couldn't be a hand. It had to be something else, a purse, a toddler, the flap of a rain jacket. But the touch sent delicious goose bumps up my spine because the possibility of a hand there one day was exciting, and I'd started to think about what kind of guy that would be.

Then a real hand clamped down on my left shoulder. I gasped with no sound and glanced up to a shadowy figure of a man so tall I could only see the outline of his face. He reached up into my white short shorts and slid his warm hand under my underwear. I stopped breathing. His fingers pushed up inside of me. My immediate reaction had been to snap my legs shut like scissors. In trying to crush him out, I fastened him in. I let that man fish around on that long ride up. I kept silent. My free hand, my fighting hand, stayed limp, my camera dangling from it.

At the top, my mother rounded us up for a picture.

"What's wrong, honey? You're all pale. Do you feel sick?"

"No, it was stuffy in there."

"Stop being such a wimp," my brother Peter teased, jabbing at me.

"Yeah," echoed the youngest, Alex, "stop being such a wimp." In the photo, my brothers are making silly faces, holding up peace signs. I am a statue. Beyond us, the lights of dusk spread across the city as far as we could see, small blinks to far and further countries I had never been to.

The aftermath was simple. I planned to make myself as ugly and fat as possible. I went back to middle school where kids were now kissing each other and instead, I grew a thick forest of rationality up around me. There was no need to tell anyone. Worse things had happened to people. I had not been raped.

When I became an official teenager, my fate of being born into a beautiful family became an irritation. No one ever called me ugly. My mother's older brother, Lauren's father, and his young family were our closest set of kin, the cool and gorgeous city people, the ones who sang "2 Legit 2 Quit" in the car and took us to restaurants where the owners knew them. They, in their homespun glamour, scooped me up with big love arms. Family was a singular devotion, and as family, we were in. Behind my braided hair and smile, though, I sensed a competitive undercurrent in their community: good looks were important. By observation, I came to see myself in the "not hot" category. In some ways, this positioning would set the framework for almost every decision I made onward. Someone needed to be the social example to prove to everyone that beauty was as empty as spun sugar. Love me anyway. I decided to not give my parents (or my extended family or the world) the pleasure and satisfaction of having a beautiful daughter. I didn't write this down in a journal, speak it aloud, or even think it in those exact words.

I just acted it out.

I did not understand this act was a violent one.

I did not understand I was violating myself by cutting myself off from pleasure and beauty and delight.

There was so much violence brewing in me.

Some people grow up with chaos and survive by creating order.

Some people grow up witnessing a false sense of order and choose to blow the system apart to extract some remnant of truth.

I was the latter.

When my father suggested I eat fewer cheese sandwiches, I asked why. Dairy was my protein; I didn't like meat. He explained cheese had a lot of fat in it, and so did hummus even though everyone thinks hummus is so healthy. Watch out for that sneaky hummus. He didn't mention any of this to my brothers. Girls at school had begun to talk about how celery was a great snack because it had negative calories. I was aware of the girl-food destiny—not yet involved with it, though. I glanced down at my scrawny body and was able, just barely, to connect that he was telling me this because he, like so many people, had his own issues with overeating and was scared for me. He continued to explain the nutritional facts. I went to the cupboard and pulled down the bread. I sliced double the amount of cheese. I pretended to listen as my knife slathered mustard all over four, instead of two, slices of bread. In minutes, I had a double sandwich. When he was done explaining, I stared at him, took a huge bite of my massive cheese sandwich, and walked out of the kitchen.

Puberty squeezed on my ribcage.

Where was my heart?

Where were my trees?

My body morphed from a playful comrade into something to hate. Even when I felt glad about what genetics had given me, I knew I was expected, as a girl, to not love my body. *Every* girl has body issues. *Every* girl wishes she looked different. These were the American world's beliefs. This was how girls connected with each other. Find the wrong thing and fix it. As much as I had vowed to be ugly and fat, I didn't actually *want* to be those things. My thighs touched when I stood with my feet together. This detail became my thing. How could I get my thighs not to touch?

Meanwhile, at church, my mother and I stood in wooden pews and sang "One Bread, One Body," the song that made us both cry a little. But I was now onto the priests, listening hard and elbowing my mother when one of them talked about people who were right (us) and people who were wrong (everyone else). She agreed with me on the injustice but held her ground. The land of the lapsed Catholics was not far away and we would both travel there. Each time we stood for communion and ate the body of Christ, I couldn't believe people around me actually took the thin tasteless wafer to be the real body, and, as I knelt in prayer, my thoughts would tumble over themselves until I ended up stranded and alone on a pile of debris wondering why we were praying over a man's body. Didn't every person come out, actually, from a woman's body? Where were the women, what about Eve, the snake, what the hell?

My body had become an aberration to me.

For the later part of middle school, I attended bar or bat mitzvah parties every weekend. This process forced a certain level of grooming. My mother bought me a pink taffeta dress. I remember how she uttered the word *taffeta* as she stroked the material. For her, it was fun to shop for the dress that would carry me through these events. But when my well-meaning mother pressed a dress or outfit against my frame, my throat closed off. The humiliation and pain was so acute I stared at the wall to keep it at bay. I became a grump who couldn't shake the underbelly. We were little people trying to act like big people. Girls took note on who was better and why. I became a second-class citizen. No boy would choose me—the freckled, brown-haired, shy girl—to dance. Could I skip this part and just be a woman?

So I let my mother choose my dress.

It was too much energy to engage in the choosing.

Once, in the middle of the dance floor, my pretty blond friend told me her boyfriend had broken up with her. He happened to also be my crush, a boy beyond my league. I clutched her into a hug as she wept into my shoulder. She smelled of tears and sweat, a smell so sensual I wanted it all over me. I was the chosen one to help her navigate this devastation. This intimacy, this connection, was a drug. We hobbled over to the chairs in the corner so we could have some privacy to discuss. I could feel the eyes of my other friends on me, all of my friends, because I was friends with everyone—the cool kids, the nerds, the middles. I couldn't bear seeing someone rejected, so always invited the outcasts to my birthday parties, and therefore had a string of followers around school. But my loyalty, truly, lay here, with the girl whose beauty so astounded me I trailed around after it in a haze.

I couldn't be the pretty one.

I could be the wise one.

For me, they became mutually exclusive.

I toned my essence so far down my core began to disintegrate.

We moved to a swamp for my high school years.

The land was made of orange groves and fireworks. It was strange, this Florida place. I was a complete stranger to myself. It was easy to hide behind homework and good grades and late-night volleyball practice, and being told over and over I was one of the best athletes. A deep sadness had taken root within me. I had not wanted to move. I didn't know who I was. To cope, I blocked my parents out of my life. My brothers, though, were allowed in my room. They would pump iron or just talk to me as I did my homework and the leafy trees outside flopped around in the wind. The company was welcome. They knew me best. They trusted my opinion. Peter would strut up to the mirror and ask me whether his muscles were getting bigger. Alex would lie in bed with me, his head on my shoulder.

"We tell you everything and you tell us nothing," they often said.

I told everyone nothing. I hoped a teacher would notice when I lounged around like Ophelia in between classes, but no one ever did. Life had channeled me toward deep navy waters, where part of me floated and part of me drowned. We were all out there, but few of us knew to look around for others. Most of me valued my own melancholy—it made me "wise." My teenage body dove and rolled for volleyballs. I slapped my teammates five. We leapt into each other's arms. But I had begun to shut down to movement. The space between my hips was a void. When I crouched on the court, the words *You are fat, You are ugly, You are fat, You are ugly* rumbled through me and, at some point, the message made it to my body and my body said, Okay, I guess I'm fat and ugly and I'd better sit down.

Nature resurrected me once.

On a weeklong school canoe trip, we slid through mangrove tunnels and spiders fell into my shirt and I learned how to breathe through my fear of them. A hard paddle across a bay in a storm made me want more, and the sight of the moon *and* the sun in the same sky made me throw my arms open. My classmates were astonished at my exuberance. I had never been in the wild. My body, for a short instant, became a body of possibilities and capacity and knowing. I wanted to learn about snakes and read constellations. Wasn't I made of stars? Weren't we all? I didn't want to dress my body up. I wanted to undress it, to get to the oldest part of who I was.

Good girls, however, do not undress.

Years later I would read about animal body and feel at home.

Hello, old friend.

You, at last.

But then it was just a glimpse.

Back in my regular world, on my sixteenth birthday, my family gathered around the cake. In front of everyone, my mom nudged me and mocked that I had probably never been kissed, right, right, right? She must have seen the wall shut down over my face. She must have wanted to take back her words.

But it was too late.

My not yet being kissed, I assumed, was because something was wrong with me. When my mother had reached toward me to say she just wanted me to feel beautiful, I heard, *You aren't beautiful.* Driving became my savior. As a responsible young woman, I ran a carpool business for the kids who lived faraway from school like us. My car also allowed me to leave and go anywhere on my own. My summer plan would have been to dress like a man—shave my head, tape my breasts—and drive across the country. I told my mother and friends so. I was adamant about the need to disguise myself. A young woman, after all, couldn't do it alone, not because she lacked strength but because the world was made of asshole men. If only I could feel the freedom a man does. If only I could pummel my way down the highway out of here to an open space.

Instead, I drove to Walgreens.

One night, I lied to my mother and told her I needed tampons. Was I really going to do this? I walked up and down carpeted aisles for half an hour and finally selected a box of devil's food cake cookies. The teller didn't seem shocked as I slid him my earned carpool cash. Maybe he was pretending not to notice how fat I was, how out of control, how ugly.

I made sure to ask for a plastic bag.

I strolled out of there with my most casual stroll.

Back in the safety of a car parked facing a ditch, I tore the box open and started with one until the cookies were gone. In the evening light, my eyes blank over concrete and palm trees, I knew I had just initiated a habit that could be with me for the rest of my life—sneak eating. Lauren and I had done it with crackers once. But that was together. You do this now, alone, and it's going to be impossible to break it later. I folded the box into the size of a wallet and wrapped it in the plastic bag. Out of my car, I leaned in and pretended to be rummaging around for old trash to throw out. Found a few gum wrappers. Walked over to the trash can and let it all go together.

No evidence.

My struggle with food as balm began.

It was easier to disassociate from my body and be defiant at the same time. It would take me years to rediscover an authentic appetite.

By then, high school was almost over.

I would be going to the University of Notre Dame. Why there? The students did community service and seemed connected to a complex world beyond college. I liked to do *the right thing*. Somehow I had worn a silver cross around my neck for four years out of duty. It may also have had to do with pleasing Pat-Pat. She, the most eager student, was the only person in her family who had never graduated from college. For two years she attended a Chicago college until her father lost his job as an owner of a car dealership. She had to forgo finishing to work at the telephone company and eventually married and had four kids. Instead of pursuing the life of an intellectual, she found ways to mother and take classes on Japanese, the Bible, Jesuits. Her oldest friend, my godmother, chose not to marry and went on to a dynamic and global career with the State Department. My mother always wondered whether her mother wanted to be a mother at all.

Before I left for college, Pat-Pat asked to speak with me.

She grabbed on to my arm and pulled me close to her face.

The tears.

"I'm proud of you, Molly. I never got to finish college. I never got to finish college," she stuttered, and it seemed she wanted to go on, to tell me the story, the why, but then she couldn't.

It was too much for her.

I didn't know how to react.

I gave her a hug and when it seemed appropriate to leave, I walked fast out of there, away from the deep pain of what hadn't happened for her, from the pain of being a trapped woman.

Going to a Catholic university didn't last long for me.

Late at night, I wrote email missives to my high school English teacher about the backward mid-century dynamics between men and women there. My lovely women friends made me laugh. We kicked and punched out to Tae Bo in our small rooms. We could go deep. But no one cared for books the way I did; no one walked down the hallway reading, no one but the seniors in my Mark Twain literature class. I was the only one in my two-hundred-person dorm who didn't go to church and most women seemed to get drunk multiple times a week. Under red maple trees on the quad, I read about women and body and shame. It wasn't hard to link that triangle to

Catholicism. I bumped into female shadows everywhere. They were everywhere.

My roommate planned to be a virgin until marriage.

"That sounds hard, and sort of strict," I said.

"Yeah, but . . ." she responded. One night, she came home drunk with her dress turned inside out and told me the boy had wanted to give it to her "the other way" to maintain her pureness. I put her to bed with a pit in my stomach. Stroked her forehead until she fell asleep. Watched the fluorescent streetlights outside until morning came. Maybe I was prude. Maybe some of this happened at every college.

The men scared me.

I wouldn't let anyone touch me. Not that anyone tried. I made myself untouchable. Beneath my frozen water flowed the rage I wouldn't be able to acknowledge for years. Alone, in my bed, in the dark, I sourced my own sexuality and soon understood how vast and unknown it was to me, and how badly I wanted to know it. My dreams took over, dreams about blood and shit, overflowing bathrooms, menstrual blood clogged in drains, my own blood running down my legs, shit smeared on every toilet I wanted to use, so much of it, this feeling I couldn't escape the mess.

Only it wasn't a mess. It was the humility of what it means to be a body. These dreams would never leave me. They would show up at points in my life when I wrestled with myself, my shape, when my body was preparing to take a deeper plunge.

Menstrual blood and shit.

Those would become my signs.

After the long vacant sad passage from girl to woman, I craved the corporeal.

Let me know what it means to embody.

After my freshman year, I decided to transfer out of there. In the packing and sorting, I failed to remember my mother's father had allowed her to go to a college only as far as a tank of gas. But she bolted after her sophomore year, left an all-girls school for a coed one. She too wanted to expand herself.

Float

The water splashes up and over.

Eula wants to splash all the water out of the bathtub and onto my mom's wooden floor. We want to rock our small boat.

"Come here, you goose," I say, and sway her body through the water toward me. This is the third place we've lived since Eula was born just over a year ago now. We take many baths together in this large claw-foot tub, now that we are back at my parents' place. Early June and we have found shelter again in our yurt.

It has canvas walls. It is a tent.

Temperature cannot be regulated.

I've tried to maintain the rhythm for Eula, by keeping her in her crib. But the yurt becomes a sauna during the day. I rock her to sleep in a room so hot she sweats through her pajamas. When night comes, cold brings her back out and into our bed. I've learned not to freak out about this. I've learned nothing stays the same: ebb and flow. We sleep on a mattress on the floor with Bru's nose pressed on our foreheads and Eula's dough love body in the middle. In the morning, we snuggle and then I load my girl into a red wagon, along with any laundry and items for the day, and we walk along the creek, under magical trees, birdsong, toward my parents' cabin. They have agreed to let us use their bathroom, as long as we move into our own house, down the field, by end of summer.

Our home is currently a shed structure covered in wood. We are all waiting for the windows to go in—usually they go in before this stage, but for a thousand reasons it had to happen in this order. My father walks down the driveway every day, can barely contain his enthusiasm, stands beneath fluttering cottonwoods, waiting. Chris is so saturated by the building process. Eighteen apertures hold no glimmer for him. He laughs at us, reminds us that windows don't mean the house is done.

For the rest of us, windows are everything.

I hover with anticipation. Once we move into our house, surely, then, I will become a steady woman, though I'm less and less sure she's a possibility in anyone. Pots and pans in one place; clothes in a dresser; a corner for a writing desk; space to be a family. I am aware of the trouble with expecting the changing circumstances of my life to change me. Doesn't prevent me from doing it anyway.

Eula glances up at me and then holds still in the bath. A few air bubbles rise and with them a little poop. I watch her with neutrality.

"Oh, there's your poop," I say.

We look together, then stand up and step out.

~

We make our way home from a Sunday barbecue, along dirt roads, the air warm and green, slow, pleasant. Alfalfa quivers in the breeze. My uterus feels heavy, a day or so away from bleeding. My peaked hormones put me on an edge. I drive through scenery people dream of and Chris and I whisper about nothing and everything as Eula sleeps. He doesn't put a hand on my leg or tucked on the brim of my pants like he used to and I don't put a hand on the back of his neck like I used to. I've recently suggested more couples therapy, but he convinces me out of it because we don't have the funds. Okay, well he could go to therapy solo, so he feels supported. I am trying to support him but he doesn't see it that way. No, he'd rather use the money and time to adventure in the mountains which is more nourishing to him, he says, than talking to someone. As we drive, though, our talk isn't about that. We argue about something I won't remember later and, as our car crests a hill surrounded by sky and green and mountains, we become two parts of a steam engine about to explode. How can the ether be so dense suddenly? My teeth are getting ground down. So are his. I call up what therapy has taught us—the importance of speaking a person's words back so you truly hear and the person knows you heard. Of course, all I'm thinking about is how *I* need to be heard. I ask him to reflect back what I said to him.

"No," he says.

I have heard him say no so many times.

I cannot bear to hear no anymore.

The heat starts at my seat, moves up fast, heart pounds, fire out my hands, keep them still, keep myself still, but the heat pulses and pressure builds, and my fear uncurls, wakes up again, beats wings hard, and when we come down the road toward our home, my glass self shatters.

I stop the car short of our driveway and start to bang on the steering wheel.

"Stop, Molly," he says with a calm voice.

I cannot bear to hear *stop* anymore. I don't stop. He gets out of the car and I crawl over the seat, reach out the window, grab at him to hold him down, but he unbuckles Eula and walks away with her. Okay, that's it. I turn the car around and prowl, follow him, tell him *Don't you dare.* He walks away, cradle-arm over Eula, protector father good father bad mother. Away. Away. I get out. I stomp to the woods and throw rocks at the ground until my body falls, pounds on grass and dirt. Give my rage back to Mama Earth like I'm supposed to. Direct it in the right direction, to a place that can hold and transmute it. Do the right fucking thing. None of it feels strange. I have been here before, many times, many moons, many ways.

But he stands at the edge of the woods and watches.

I don't want to be watched.

That changes everything.

"You are ruining me," I scream at him, over and over again, my arms punching the air between us, until there is no sound from my chest anymore. I want to scream, *You man.* My head hangs until I glance up and Eula has awoken. She stares at me, groggy, unsure of what has happened. What is her mama doing over there, why does she have claw marks on her face, why is her body on the ground?

My body responds to her.

I stand. I breathe. I walk toward her. I notice owls in a tree. They are all calling me back. Come back, Mama. Come back.

Later, Chris will call it "The Event" and say he forgives me but it can never happen again. I won't have any energy to have a conversation about it. The morning after, as sun pours into our yurt, I utter an urgent prayer. Please lead me to health. Now. I cannot lose them. I cannot lose myself.

~

Holcomb asks whether my rage comes before my menses. She wants to run a test.

"Is it all the time or tied to your cycle?"

"Probably. The day before I bleed I seem to go insane."

She explains that our doctor-culture name of PMS can be misleading. It *is* a chartable hormonal shift in the body, but there is a deeper level. What has been buried will come to the surface during this time. When people write a woman off as being *hormonal*, they dismiss her and make her feelings sound irrational. She should not dismiss the feelings. Though rage feelings are magnified feelings, they are real.

"Don't discount that," she says.

~

What I learn: Women and snakes. Long history. Our power is often graceful, coiled up and ready at our root. Not meant to be tamped down. But also not meant to flare and flare and flare without purpose. As a young woman, I saw enough unexpressed women to make me never want to be unexpressed. Pregnancy awoke my deep anger. I would not let anyone silence it. Do not hold me down. Do not tell me how not to be. Do not tell me what not to say. There's been enough of that already. Beneath it was a great sadness. An enraged woman is unexpected and, therefore, a horror.

I gave myself permission to be her.

I gave myself permission to flare it up.

No more well-behaved woman for me.

It continued.

It has become repeated anger, the kind that loops and loops, over and over again. It leads to heart problems. It overworks the amygdalae and adrenals. It pauses the growth of new neurons. It becomes a pattern. It can be hard to shake. But the worst part: rage can sever all other feelings so you forget you were *also* joyful.

Joy.

There has always been joy within me.

Do not forget that. Go excavate it.

It occurs to me traditional cultures are/were, by design, a postpartum support group. Mothers walked to gather with other mothers at a market or field or other home. They talked, worked, laughed, sang, and grieved together. Their older children played nearby and the bigger ones instructed the little ones on the ways of life. The baby stayed strapped to a mama or got passed around to other women. If a woman needed to rest, the other women took on her extra work. It was a cycle. I don't mean to glorify it. I only mean to say it is anathema to even want that today. We expect a partner to meet most of our needs. That does not make sense. That does not make sense on the most primal of levels. In constant community, I suspect normal rage would signal a person to pay attention, process and feel the grief, and then dance into pleasure. We would learn the art of moving between light and dark—not getting stuck in one.

Rage on top of rage creates more rage.

I've made so much space for my rage.

I want to welcome back my joy.

I want to make contact with my joy.

I've elbowed it out.

~

A few days later, we end up at a wedding. We stand outdoors watching Chris's navy-pilot cousin get married in Montana. People calculate the perfect weekend to achieve the green glory no one realizes only lasts for two months here. They've found it today. I've always seen marriage as a courageous journey where you get to witness and be witnessed. What connection. What potential for love. I grab for my husband's hand. We are changed but the same somehow.

I never thought I'd become this kind of middle-aged woman.

I want to stop the show and start a group conversation: yep, that vow is for real, yeah, and that one is really hard.

We left Eula to sleep over with my parents in the hallway of their cabin. We'll return and sleep on the daybeds because it's too complicated to get to the yurt in the dark with an already-slumbered babe. All should be well. I nursed her before leaving and will nurse her when we return. Because I didn't have anything appropriate to wear for black-tie or because I didn't make the time to find anything, my mother's clothes came to the rescue—again. They smell of her perfume from years ago. It exacerbates me to be draped in my mother, not myself. I look like I'm going to a funeral, in all black with a sequin top as the only shimmer. I would prefer feathers. Chris's uncle keeps calling me a black widow spider. Tease, tease. He must sense my venom.

I allow myself to get swept up in the love.

My quiet mother-in-law leaps up and dances with the groom because his mother passed away from a brutal cancer years ago. She awes me with this move, to step out of her comfort zone with such grace. The whole ceremony and celebration transports me to a space away from what has been.

My takeaway: It's crucial to get out and away.

When the band starts, I dart to the dance floor without thinking, because dancing at weddings is what I love, what *we* love. When I hit my first bounce-hip move, pee floods out of me and as everyone else accelerates, I slow down, and my hips go stuck as I waddle back to a wall. Slip out to the bathroom without anyone seeing me. I can smell the sagebrush at night. Damp sagebrush. The mountains hum behind me, dark shadow shapes, like old grandmothers watching everyone below. Under these stars, the wrecking ball presses on my chest as I lean over a wooden fence. C'mon. C'mon. I cannot drag Chris into this. I gulp and tell myself that *this*, along with Eula, are the reasons I must heal my pelvic floor.

I have to be able to dance.

I have to be able to dance with her.

Acceptance is avoidance. It's been over a year. I thought by now . . . I don't know what I thought. Do more Kegels. Do more. Fix yourself even though you're tired and the whole process exhausts you.

I never go back to dance.

We walk toward the car, arm in arm, under moon, stars, open western sky, some part of the old us awakened. He has doe eyes. My breasts are engorged and they hurt. We climb into our gray hatchback.

"You have to get this milk out of me," I say to Chris in the dark.

"Really?" he asks. "Are you serious?"

"Yes, now, get on there and suck it out."

We both laugh, but I'm serious. There is nowhere to hand-express my milk and it wouldn't be fast enough anyway. I lift my shirt, snap off my bra, and there goes his head, ducked under, as people walk behind our parked car in the dark to their cars. Look at us, doing this thing in the car. Think of all the teenage boys who would give anything to do this to a woman in a car.

"You have to *really* suck hard, babe," I explain.

"It's so sweet," he gurgles up. "I didn't expect that."

"Major nutritional value," I tell him, and we hunker down some more so no one sees us. A few minutes later, I have some relief. But before he latches onto the next one, he pauses.

"Hold on, I need a break. This is hard work. My jaw hurts."

We finish and laugh the whole way home, across the valley, speculating on which of our guy friends we think may or may not have tasted breast milk. One day, nursing will become a thing of the past for me. I don't know when; not soon, though. It has been the one easy and heavenly—and that isn't a word I use—ritual in the last year.

Later that night, while Chris and Eula sleep, I grab my own re-engorged breast and put my mouth to it. My large breasts come in handy here. Beloved breasts. In the clear moonlight, I suck out my own sweet milk.

It doesn't seem strange at all.

~

In my dream, I fly a paper plane made of lavenders and blues and oranges. I have aviator goggles on and am a teacher of planes. But I crash into a lake and come up, gasping for air, yelling, "Help, help!" There is a man on a paddleboard. I am expecting him to come help but, in a flash, I know I can help myself. My screams stop. I follow the river of feathers and swim to that far-away shore.

~

The windows could sweat. It is ninety-five degrees, a hot sun, never thick here, just burning. We retreat to my parents' cool bedroom of teal concrete floors and dark blue pillows. Eula rolls around on the bed, for once okay with not being outdoors. She usually pounds on the door, wants out, like a dog. Naked. Where she can pee on the grass, or on the plastic toilet we've put out there for her. The porch gives her tiny splinters on her bum, but she doesn't seem to mind. I like to watch our bare feet touch the grassy muddy earth together. Yesterday we sat on the warm stone. She pulled at her vulva and opened her other hand in question.

This is how we communicate.

This is how she asks me questions.

"That's your vulva," I explained. "Like Mama."

She nodded.

Now she turns and slides off the bed to rummage through Mare's scarves in the chest. She insists, by pointing, on wearing purple pajamas and a black-and-white striped dress with a scarf in her hair. We oblige, help her fit her baby legs into the pants. She gazes at herself in the mirror with the seriousness of an actor, and then laugh laugh laughs. We've been grooming together for the past few months— brushing hair and teeth as we sing. Eula watched a friend show me some yoga postures. Ever since then, when I push back into downward dog, she walks around me, pushes on my lower back, touches my feet, then my knees, as if she is positioning me. Then she flops down into a pose herself.

"Oh-p," is what we say together when anything happens. How is it possible to have staring contests that end in peals of laughter with a one-year-old? I never knew children are so *themselves* the moment they arrive.

Language.

I can hear the language train approaching from a distance. Here it comes.

She gestures to everything and then asks me, with a nod of her head, to repeat the name for it. On her crib in the yurt, the "knot in the wood" is a favorite to repeat. Something about the word "knot" sends her off into uncontrollable giggles.

After our dress-up day in Mare's room, we stroll down to the yurt. My mom stands on the porch and waves. Eula waves back as I pull her red wagon through our mowed grass pathway and we say good night to the cottonwoods, the creek, the owls. I pull the drape around her crib, unroll the canvas blinds, and she burrows into my clothes drawer. The hour before bed allows us to get any excess energy out. When I turn around to scoop her up, she tosses a few shirts at my feet and points at my chest.

"You want me to put these on?" I ask.

She nods and then steps a few feet back. She cocks her head to watch. I slip down to my bra and pull a black flowered shirt over my head. She smiles and then tosses another one to me. Are we doing this? I realize my daughter is dressing me, somehow telling me it's okay to dress myself. Five shirts later, she nuzzles up to me, rubs her eyes, and we are done, but some old self within is saying, *Let's do more, let's do this all the time,* this *is fun.*

~

On our drive back from town one afternoon, Eula coos out at cows in the backseat. I tell my mom about my recent action plan. I need to cut gluten and dairy out of my diet in order to truly heal my thyroid. They are inflammatory foods.

"And god knows I'm inflamed enough," I laugh, and she laughs with me.

"Well, you just have to do it then," she says.

"I know, but it's hard," I say, and then hedge whether to share more, to expose what food dredges up in me, why it's not as simple as just *saying sayonara*, as Pat-Pat would say. I no longer want to trim my mother out of my emotional life with my precise X-Acto blade. My mom knows food can be my drug, but she doesn't experience it for herself. I've never seen the woman overeat a day in her life, and not because she's restricting. She eats everything in moderation—such color and balance on her plate every meal. No one thinks her to be a smoker because she doesn't smell of smoke, but cigarettes are her challenge. Soon, though, she will let them go after decades of counting on them.

"It's strange to say it," I start, "but gluten and dairy are my only reliable friends. I mean, that's what it feels like, anyway. Bread and cheese."

"I get it," she laughs. "I feel the same way about cigarettes."

"Yeah?" I say.

"I even wrote a letter to the tobacco gods once."

We are more similar than I think.

~

On a dry, baked, rocky ascent, I watched Holcomb fling her daughter onto her back so easily, side hip, bend, scoot her to the back, and draw up the straps of the carrier. No need for another person to help. No extra stuff. No hat. No sunscreen. I haven't seen this easy maneuver of hers before. She's always had her daughter on her back by the time we arrive. By contrast, I could have been embarking on a desert expedition with Eula in a bulky framed backpack, my huge straw hat, globs of sunscreen, long-sleeve shirt, bottle of water.

I thought I could injure myself if I move in ways I used to.

It cannot be true.

Later, I practice once and then strap Eula to my back in the carrier.

We step out the door and seek shade.

I don't wear anything but a tank, a skirt, and my daughter. I don't want to hide my body anymore. We walk with Bru through the woods, grass grazing arms, and then, at last, arrive under the treed canopy of the creek. The water runs coppery and low over rocks in July, when farmers use it to irrigate their fields. I step in, welcome the cold water to my feet.

We move upstream.

Rustle in the willows. A fawn darts by, up and over the bank and away.

"A baby deer," I say to Eula. "Did you see?"

I don't care if I pee all over myself—into this water. Eula leans over the carrier and peers into shade and sun on water. We crawl over fallen cottonwoods. We balance on rocks. We slip and then don't on slippery stones. We dip her baby feet in the flowing water. We move all the way up the creek, as far as we can go on this land.

It feels good to move my body with abandon.

It feels like a baptism.

As water rushes over my feet, I call up my thousands of agile moments. Must be able to see them to make them real again.

I *am* made of healthy tissue.

I am made of healthy tissue. We, Eula and I, are made of healthy tissue.

I must repeat this over and over and over and over and over and over and over and over and over and over and over and over and over and over and over and over and over and over and over and over as water rushes over and over and over and over me.

~

What I learn: No one has personally ascribed any of my story to me. My shovel can only dig so deep. I have recently considered a jade egg. It is a practice from four thousand years ago in China, supposedly taught only to the queen and concubines. Though many believed the result— tight sexual organs—was to please the king, it actually improved the woman's health and her connection to spirit. The egg gives a woman a felt-sense of where and how her muscles work together to lift up the Chi. As a woman tones, her orgasms become longer lasting and more intense and she has a stronger sexual flow, and therefore, perhaps more important, a stronger divine flow within her. Without that strength, you leak urine *and* life force. Once again, who knew? Years ago, Chris made me a wooden oval for that purpose. Neither of us knew much about vaginal weight lifting but he was tapping into a knowing beyond him. Here, tend to your femaleness. I wish I had. Instead of the egg, I buy what a friend recommends for mother-vaginas: Lelo beads. But they seem to push my prolapse out, so I stop and decide to push past my fear of an egg doing the same and try one, one day, some day.

~

Eula tucks her cold feet between my legs. I open my eyes to a flaxen dawn. It settles on the yurt's wooden floor, and the sound of a hawk and the creek comes into focus. My body snuggles us both back, closer to Papa.

"Come closer," I whisper to Chris. "Keep us warm."

My words wake her up.

Once she's up, she's up, but we try to lure her back.

"Come play, come yank on our ears," I beg as she prances around.

"Come do *anything* but get up," Chris moans, and flops a heavy arm over me. But my firebird is ready for the day, and it happens to be the day of my birth.

I've written notes to both my parents. It's my turn to honor them for making me and raising me. My father will get on a plane and move to New York for work today. He'll come back to visit, but not to live, not until he can. I'm surprised by my whole-body sadness about it. Somehow it feels like the end of a hard era, one I want to commemorate by taking a picture of us all in front of the cabin, frame it—*The Year(s) We Cohabitated and Molly Went Loca.*

We walk into a cabin full of balloons.

My parents blew them all up. The tears gather behind my eyes. Why is everyone so nice to me? I hug them and Eula orates and swats at each balloon. Bru makes a quick escape back to the calm porch.

Chris makes gluten-free blueberry pancakes and we all celebrate before the airport run.

I usually walk in the woods on my birthday.

We drive up to Emerald Lake and Eula demands to walk the trail on her own. She can do it on her own. She wants to do everything on her own. No hands and when she sees me strap the carrier around my waist, she pushes my leg away.

"Be mindful," I say, as she pulls herself up and over rocks. The word *careful* is too loaded. I don't want her to walk through life as a careful woman. I've heard Holcomb request *wise feet* from her daughter. This I also like and adopt. We hear a helicopter fly overhead. She pauses, lifts her finger to her ear. I hear it, Mama. I hear it, Papa. Over roots and stones, she grunts.

"Do I grunt?" I ask Chris.

"That's a May family thing," he says, and pinches me. "You *all* speak in sounds." I've recently made a point of doing cartwheels in front of Eula on the lawn. They aren't perfect. They almost rip my pelvis in half, but I can do them. I want her to know that her mama can move. This action may be a different overextension of *the mother*, but it matters to me. She stands naked in the grass and frantically signs for more, her fingers pecking together. Again, Mama, again. But now, here on the mountain, after an hour of walking/stopping/investigating, she's hit her maximum. Tired girl.

I try to load her on my back because it's a wanting-Mama-not-Papa moment. She grabs for my chest so I slide her in front; she nurses and falls asleep. I haven't carried her in a carrier on my front since she was an infant during our hikes with Holcomb, and even then not often because of the extreme pressure on my bladder.

"You sure that's okay, babe?" Chris asks.

"Yeah, it'll be fine." For the next hour, I walk downhill with a twenty-five-pound baby on my belly and somehow, I do not pee. Is it that I haven't drunk enough water today? The mourning moves in me. It isn't a wrecking ball; it's a wave. I never got to carry her this way without feeling awful and peeing. As my feet move over roots and rocks and brown earth, a resurrection begins. We arrive at the parking lot and I keep walking. We exchange the sacred parental nod that signals we want to keep our child asleep. I continue down the dirt road, aspens lean toward us, and my feet could go on forever now, one foot at once, down this road, as long as necessary, dust at my heels, dust on my toes, until the mountains greet me, and I will walk over them and to a valley and then to the ocean. I will focus on what is good and working—in my body, my marriage, my daughterhood, my motherhood.

Eula wakes to beating sun.

"Hey, sweets," I say, and wipe her sweaty brow. I turn around to beckon Chris and the car. When I hand her over to him, my lower back has gone numb. But, for the first time in fifteen months, I have held my bladder.

We drive home.

That afternoon, we walk up to the bench above our house and bury Eula's umbilical cord. I try not to think back to why we didn't do it on her birthday. Nothing but bluebird sky up here. We squint out to all the mountains, squat down together, and dig a hole in a patch of sagebrush. I show her the heart-shaped cord and she tries to pull it apart. She has no idea what we are doing but it matters to me to say it anyway.

"This," I tell her, "is where I peed on a pregnancy stick and we knew you would come to us."

I was a different woman then.

We place four stones over the cord. What does it means to cut a cord from a person—your mother, your daughter, your self? Eula might think this all strange and intense when she's a woman, or not. I don't know how she will develop. Chris hugs me from behind as Eula picks sage. I let myself fall backward into his embrace, but with caution still.

He puts his hand between my legs and breathes into my ear.

I pause.

I've wanted this moment for so long. I don't know what to do with it now. It's too much. It's almost too much to be held this way. I force myself to trust it.

He tells me he has written me a letter about why he fell in love with me.

It's too much to feel.

When we start to love-make at dusk, he stretches over me and the pressure of his body releases a flood.

"I think I peed," I sigh, and we both stroke the wet spot on our sheets.

"It's okay," he whispers, and pulls me toward him.

~

My mother looks up from her mop bucket. She's tied a red bandanna around her forehead and for some reason this makes me want to call her Rambo. The rental guests arrive at the guesthouse in an hour.

"Can I help you clean, Mom?" I ask.

"No, no, it's fine," she says and keeps moving. Eula and I wait in the cabin and try to tidy up stacks of magazines for my mom. When she gets unsettled, my brothers and I have often teased or berated her because it scares us. She is supposed to be the steady one. What I need to do is give her what I want from Chris: hug her, tell her I'm sorry it's frustrating or hard. I want to be soft with her in the way I am with Eula. My mother always put herself last.

She never got to have a mood, or an "Event."

She stomps onto the porch and waves from the window at Eula, who is now dressed in a blue ribbon and a towel around her head.

When my mother smiles, the world calms down.

We go into her bedroom and she takes out the pear-shaped ivory necklace. Ivory is layered with complexity and gray striations. Pat-Pat gave it to her for her twenty-first birthday. Where had she bought it? What thoughts had rolled through her head, her heart, as she picked it for her daughter? I have seen my mother wear this ivory on a long thin chain for years—over blouses, sweaters, at Christmas, to the movies. One day it will be mine. One day it will be Eula's. We all take turns placing it around each other's necks, like the anointed ones. I wonder how ivory changes based on who wears it. My mother uses it as her pendulum as well.

"Open your palm, Eula," my mom asks.

She does.

My mother places the ivory in her chubby little hand, and Eula nods at Mare, takes in what all of this means, as if she is telling her something about this object. How does she *know*?

~

There is a cycle. Here is how it goes. As much as I soften, when our history surfaces, the world is made of small electric shocks. Isn't this how it is with all parents and children?

Act 1—*I hurt my mother.* My mother requests we be cleaner and not leave our stuff on the daybed. I get offended and say, "Well, what do you want me to do? Put it outside." Then she explains that she loathes giving her time to cleaning but is bound to it right now. Pat-Pat made her clean banisters till they shone, never asked her brothers to do it, only her, so she hates it, there.

"You hate us being here," I tell her. We've overstayed our welcome. I know that's true. We sleep in the yurt but days require running water so we stay in the cabin and nearby. We have been in her space too long, and we're so close to being out. It's already August, Mom, only another week or so. Plus, I'm not a messy person. I never have been. We fight some more and some more.

Act 2—*Day of avoidance.* Eula and I spend much of the day under cottonwoods down by the creek stacking rocks. She is a Taurus, all earth, and, whoa, does she want earth, stones, to throw them, lay her body across them. No breeze. We cuddle up on a rock surrounded by gurgles and flowing water. That rock is who my mom is—unflappable, in general, among chaos. I scoop up a long gray stone to give to her (my attempt at reconciliation). Heat on my back. I peel off my shirt. Eula stands naked on the rock, grabs my breast, and nurses. I could do this all year long, this right here. This would be a great photo—the phrase *if I were thinner* pops up and I shoo it away. When we climb back up the bank; my mom is getting into her car and calls out to me.

"Want me to get you a big box of pads at Costco?" she asks (her attempt at reconciliation).

"No, thanks," I say, but what I mean is No, no, no, I don't want anymore humiliating *Always* Extra-Long Pads with Wings. Even though I still need them.

Act 3—*My mom hurts me.* The next day, while Eula is on a walk with Chris, my mom finds a coconut ice-cream bar wrapper in my grocery bag.

"Ah-ha, I *see*," she says, waving it in my face. "You still love that ice cream, don't 'cha?" I wasn't even trying to hide it. I'm actually not ashamed of that particular sneak eating. But my shame reaction is muscle memory. I tell her she's being mean. She says she's just teasing and tells me that she feels abused by me.

"Abused?" I say. "Now that's a strong word. You sure you want to use that word?" and as I say what I say I realize my language is abusive.

"We've all heard enough about your *troubles*," she hisses at me. "I just hope you learn how to take care of yourself. I haven't seen you do that yet."

That sets me off.

"Do you know what it feels like?" I scream. "Do you know what it feels like to be betrayed by my body? *No one* here knows what that feels like and do you know what it's like to go on a walk and pee and bleed all over yourself and on the car seat while your thyroid doesn't work, and that's become normalized for everyone, including me, but it's not normal! And I'm trying to reconcile all the complicated feelings I have about my body based on how we were raised."

"What does that mean?" she asks.

"All the messages I got about not being able to wear those pants, and blah blah blah."

"Yeah, well, Pat-Pat told me I had a big butt and always said, with her critical tone, that I had my grandmother's legs. But I don't remember ever saying anything like that to you."

"You didn't," I explain, "not exactly."

We comment on our daughter's bodies because the world commented on ours. It's an old conversation. It's proven that the less a mother makes out-loud observations about the shape and size of her daughter's body (good or bad), the less her daughter will have any judgment toward her body. It's a rope with knots and each one of us is holding on tight, even when we don't want to.

We end calm.

I leave in my car to go away and my sobs take over. An owl swoops in front of me, saying yes, it's okay, go deeper, this is hard, but you must.

My heart has cracked. Will I ever grow up?

~

On our last night in the yurt, something happens. It is the eve of moving out of my parents' space and into our own home—at long last—and a massive cottonwood tree falls over our path to the cabin. We don't hear it. There is no wind. When we wake, we say good-bye to the yurt, bless it by running our hands along the wall. This three-month yurt life with child was cozy and messy. I will miss the close togetherness. We step off our porch and amble through green grass.

"Whoa," I say.

"Whoa," says Chris, who never says *whoa*.

"Oh-p," says Eula.

Across and over the fallen tree, we see my mom waving at us.

That afternoon, as Chris hauls our clothes to the house, I watch my mother talk to the tree. She walks up and down it and her hand bump-bumps along the bark. When we join her, she says, "Do you realize that it was one trunk split into two branches and one of those branches is double-branched, like me and Dad, and the other one is a single branch, like you." Whoa, we say to each other, and marvel. My mom was never this symbolic when I was young. A medicinal smell wafts up from broken branches. Eula crunches the tiny branches and comes up sticky with orange cottonwood sap on her bare feet.

We decide to call it the Boom-ba tree, because whenever Eula falls, we say, *Boom-ba!* I saw off a large branch to put in our house. I want to be reminded of softness, of what it means to detach—cut a cord—and still love.

"It's a great omen," my mom says.

"That it is," I agree.

~

The next day, Chris makes two wooden doors for our house. Last minute. Our friends from New Zealand arrive to spend three weeks with us. We haven't seen them in years. But the timing is not ideal. We haven't had a moment to acknowledge our *home* or that Chris built it with his own hands. Concrete floors, shed roof, windows open up to the hill, a tiny room for Eula and a long steep wooden ladder that leads to a loft for us. Our bare living room becomes a sleepover party.

We go with the flow—boxes, clothes, and kitchen pots everywhere.

The house isn't done, but we can live with an unfinished bathroom and kitchen.

It's a mess, but life has been a mess.

"*You* built this," I whisper to Chris in bed. "Thank you."

Our friends make no demands. They are happy-go-lucky. After each meal, I am able to pick up Eula and navigate her sticky food hands and face and body to the sink while singing, "I want to dance with you, my girl." We do it every time. Nothing strains me about the situation or chaos, other than Chris. He is free from the house for the first time since Eula's birth. I want him to myself. I want every part of him. But my husband only has eyes for our friends, talks with them with a lightness I haven't experienced since pregnancy. He won't look at me. Suddenly the fury in me rises. What about me? What about his wife, the woman who has been waiting her daughter's entire life to have some time with her husband? We've always had a deep friendship. At least before all of this. I want it back. I want him back. I expected the hardship to evaporate when we moved into the house.

But I say nothing—my new practice is to pause, not react. It's okay, viper. Settle down. None of this is permanent. Keep your eyes peeled for the joy. For a few days, this works. Then, under a hot sweltering sun, Chris and I stand outside alone before I leave for a meeting.

"We might go exploring on Saturday," he says, and the high lilt of his voice gives away that he's nervous about what he's saying.

"Just you two?" I ask.

"Yeah, we can 'hoon around a bit then," he says, using Kiwi slang and what he means is that the men can adventure and not be held back by the women and children. I know he needs it. I know it is really what he wants more than anything—time away from a domestic world, time for play in the mountains and no strained conversation, time to unwind from this challenging last few years. Of course he would rather do that than be with me, or include me. I do get it. As I stare at burnt-out grass, though, my chest still stings. Wish he would say: "I'm going to go on this adventure, and when I return, I can't wait to go on an adventure with you." He won't ever say that. I've already asked for that introductory phrase—for years. Wish he would prioritize me in his orbit.

"Okay," I say, and turn my body away from his. "So, for our first free weekend in over a year, I get to stay home and play house."

"*Molly*, you don't have to stay home. You all can go on your own adventure with the kids. They are visiting us from across the world. I have to make time for him."

"But not for me, never for me."

"What do you want me to do?"

I recognize the impossibility. I'm being an ass.

"I don't care anymore. Do whatever," I say, and I walk toward my car without a goodbye and the awful satisfaction of being the one who leaves. At least I walked away. What would it be to be free? Mountains and cows and alfalfa fields and I have no response to any of it. Nature doesn't have a place anymore. Sobs taper off and get replaced by cold and reckless calculation. I never thought I would be this woman. I need to do something drastic. My hands test the wheel. Small car wobbles as it careens down the road. Crows rest on fence posts. If I crash before town, no one else will be hurt out here in the country. Then he'll know my pain and have to look into my eyes, even if they are dead eyes, and care.

I can make this happen with one turn of the wheel.

Eula.

My Eula-babes.

Thoughts of her bring me back into my heart and the sobs crowd out the cold calculation again. I pull over and call a friend.

"Hey, Molls." I didn't expect her to answer.

"Hey."

"What's wrong?"

"I almost crashed my car."

"Where are you?"

"Pulled over."

"Tell me what happened."

"I fuck everything up."

She talks me down from believing I have ruined everything for my family. I thank her. She makes me promise to call her every hour until I'm home with Chris.

On my way home, the mountains try to help. Rise up with us. We are cold. We are also green. We understand your man. We also understand you. Everything erodes. Everything is made again. Nothing is as big as it seems. Even we aren't as big as you see us. I hear them but don't listen. My plan becomes disconnection. It is the safest plan. Just disconnect from him and go into autopilot. As I stuff clothes into the washing machine, he comes up behind me and pulls me into a long embrace. This is how he gets when he feels he's done the right thing. I can tell he must know something. My friend called Chris who called Holcomb and they have triaged. He knows not to involve my parents because I don't go there with them. We must start to monitor me more carefully. It's a *we* now, he says. I have been heard by my husband. Holcomb tells me to please feel free to tell her what I'm feeling—*any* time. I haven't been responsible to myself, or to her. I've assumed I can handle it. The neurotransmitter test results are back. We meet at her office. My serotonin levels are actually fine. A general antidepressant might have helped a small bit, and I did consider it, but it would not have addressed the entire picture. I would have continued to flounder.

They say it gets worse before it gets better.

This is a cultural black hole. We do not take care of our women, especially our mothers. If a woman with a mood shift after birth actually admits to it, she finds herself under the catchall label *postpartum depression.* It is not always accurate. Some women weep. Some women rage. Some women go blank. Some women cannot shake anxiety. We are nuanced creatures. We don't fit one category. Depression doesn't always look like what we think depression looks like.

Couldn't the name be, instead, *postpartum challenge?*

Maybe more women would seek help then.

Less shame around that language.

It's clear I've been having a postpartum challenge. I don't doubt that. I'm not ashamed of it, just trying to understand the physical part from the emotional part from the circumstantial part. How do they affect each other? The ecosystem of my body is complex. The test reveals my norepinephrine has skyrocketed off the charts—fight or flight, rage, irritability. My GABA is also low—overwhelmed and overstimulated. Holcomb prefers not to give a static diagnosis but suggests I might have PMDD, premenstrual dysphoric disorder, linked to my menstrual cycle and exacerbated by the thyroid piece. My menstrual charts track that my car-crash reaction and "The Event" both happened a few days before my bleeding. Of course. Why couldn't I have seen that and responded accordingly? We talk about supplements and hormone replacement. She suggests I start to wean Eula so we have more options for herbs, and drugs, if I'm open to that. There is also the additional possibility that the hormones in my system, from nursing, are affecting my moods.

I don't want to wean my baby at eighteen months. But so I begin.

~

What I learn: The sea change washes toward me. Premenstrual syndrome is actually not a malady but a signal. The dark pulse of it lets us know when to start the retreat away from responsibility. Responsibility, in our modern world, means schedules, long workdays, anything that maxes or stresses us out. Only we don't *ever* retreat. Both women and men have been taught that to take downtime is weak. Continue on, instead. But we miss out. Ideally, menstruation is a time to renew, clear the calendar and create a sanctuary. What few know is that our potential for insight and divine connection while bleeding is amplified. Pliny said a menstruating woman could break mirrors, sour wine, rust iron, dull knives. He may have cast it as a negative spoken out of his fear, but he saw the power. Our female body is connected to source. When we miss this rich window, our PMS gets misdirected and our female power sabotages itself. Month after month, we repeat. We lose the opportunity. Then we get mad about it without exactly knowing what we are mad about. We are mad at an untapped self. We are mad that there is a much deeper cultural phenomenon at play.

It isn't one woman's solitary "hormonal freak-out"—it's all of us.

Every female passes through a few hormonal gateways: first menses, childbirth (if chosen and possible), and menopause. These are opportunities to open and connect to the deepest essence within oneself, astral-plane moments where we are able to see with crystal clarity. Our body leads us there, whether we want to go there or not. It is designed to move through huge passages. We are designed for those profound shifts. But we have almost no cultural conversation about any of it.

My laboring woman didn't intellectualize this concept. She embodied it. She understood the importance of rest and pause and breath without anyone having to give her a textbook about it.

She was the living cycle. She lives in every woman. She must still live in me. She is and all women are the understory—that place where loamy soil and nutrients support the entire forest ecosystem to grow upward. Nothing could survive without her. She is the bedrock. She is all-knowing. I wonder what else we haven't acknowledged her to be. I wonder what she will be next.

~

Eula has begun to put necklaces on me. We sit on the concrete floor of our new house together and intertwine our warm legs. She chooses a strand of red cinnabar beads and anoints me with them—then the white ones, then silver. When I'm ready to move on to another activity, she pulls my arms, pulls me back down, *No, Mama,* and wants to go on for hours. I feel like a queen.

"Thank you for decorating me, sweets," I say, and she giggles.

"Can I decorate you too?" I ask.

"No-kay, *Mama*," she insists, and pushes on my chest indicating that she wants this to be a one-way street for now.

When she wakes at dawn, we snuggle on an old rattan loveseat I used to play on as a child. She nurses as the moon goes down and the sun spreads across cottonwoods. My child has honey-brown hair now because her papa and uncle and grandmother once did at this age. I stroke her head, cheeks, arms, legs—all of her. The other night she fussed and started to fake cry (it's a thing she does now) and I asked her what was wrong. Did she want to read a book together? No, she shoved it away. She crawled into my lap and hugged me and it became clear all she needed was a long, slow, uninterrupted hug from her mama. We sat that way before bed for ages. No milk. No books. No rituals. Just a hug, her body heavy on my chest, gazing out the window at trees. It doesn't seem strange to me that these holy moments can coexist with such despair. When I placed her in bed, she sunk down, satisfied, peaceful and not one little peep when I left the room. The morning time is my favorite time. It will be the last nurse session I let go of because this will be gradual over the next one to two months. But these days, a few minutes into it, she already says, as if she knows, "All done," and pulls my shirt over my breasts.

~

On the cabin's porch, I have my monthly call with my counselor Janice.

It's a quiet oasis up here, under the cottonwoods by the creek, with my mom out of town and my babe and man in town. I tell her about the norepinephrine but hear the excuse in what I'm articulating. She listens and then reminds me that the body reacts to the state of the mind.

"Honey, I'm concerned you're stuck in a rage cycle," she says softly.

"Of course I am," I say.

"Molly, you have healthy anger, honey, but I think you've also indulged in your anger," she says. The word *indulged* bludgeons my face. I don't say anything, so she continues. She tells me that anger is addictive. It may feel like power but that's only because anger lets us feel when we are depressed and unable to feel sadness. This is exactly what I've come to on my own—my attachment to anger, my dangerous replay of it, my hold on being the dark, wild woman who spits out if she needs to, even though anyone who knows me beyond close friends and family always says, "I can't imagine you enraged at all." The cure for rage isn't more anger. I must accept my rage, she says, and parent those parts of me who are raging. Then do something kind for them. She keeps talking and, though she's heard me and validated me a thousand times over, what I feel is squashed, told off, told I'm bad. I know what she says is true but I'm not ready to hear it from someone else, not this way.

I don't have ears for anyone or anything anymore.

"I don't want to be silenced by anyone, even *you*," I lash out.

"Molly," she bellows with a deep voice I've heard before when she's serious, "you are being mean. Listen to you. Listen to how mean you are being. Listen to how mean you are being."

I can't believe she is calling me *mean*.

I can't believe this is happening.

I can't be on this phone anymore.

I don't want her to know I'm crying.

I don't ever want to talk to her again.

We are silent for a minute.

"How do you feel?"

"Disconnected," I mutter.

"If you need to hang up to go cry . . ."

All I needed was permission. I hang up on her and vow to never call her again. Later she will leave me a message explaining that it was an intervention with love. She felt she had to jolt me out of my rage cycle. Rage is just energy. It's time to stop processing and tracking and just work with the energy. Move the energy *through your body*. If I don't want to work with her, that's okay, but I need to find someone immediately and start working once a week. She's concerned and says again, "Remember, honey, that rage is just an energy in your body."

My body rolls off the porch and somehow gets up to stomp around the grass, arms punch sky, stumble, stumble, what just happened, phone thrown to ground, body thrown to ground, roll down, roll around, pull at grass, more grass, cover head, cover face, cover scream, curl up, pull at grass, cover head, curl up.

~

Gray clouds. I sit in my gray hatchback three days later and call Janice. Car windows go down on a dirt road nearby a field with three horses. My ear buds go in. The only reason I call her back is because it took courage for her to name the truth and risk me leaving and some therapists would have never done so.

"I want to roar, howl, scream," I say.

"Can you put the phone down and scream? I'll wait," she asks.

"I'm too embarrassed," I say.

"That's okay."

We continue, and I ask where ritual has gone. People used to move a shadow through the body—put on a mask, dance, and sing. I want to move my body. I want to express it out. I don't want to be in love with my wounds anymore. I speak in plain language. There is no longer a place for intellect. I close my eyes as Janice speaks to me and I see a room covered with charcoal sketches of one woman's face in rage, despair, joy, shame, envy, boredom, frustration, hope, embarrassment, ecstasy, regret, gratitude, empathy, contempt, love.

Nothing has ever seemed so beautiful.

"What if feeling these feelings draws bad things to me?" I ask, even though I've already felt them.

"Create a container to feel your feelings. Feel them. Cry them. Scream them," she says. "And *then*, reclaim trust and use the law of attraction."

The last part sounds impossible.

~

In September, the fields turn yellow-white. My workshops begin. I go back to teaching other people how to own their stories while I try to own my own. After my steamy shower, Eula stands nearby to watch me put on a skirt she's never seen and arrange my hair in a new way. She takes a step back, points her hand at me, waves it up and down as if she is directing traffic, and says, "Ooooo nice, Mama."

My daughter has already healed my relationship to clothes.

When I return from my first day away, I strap Eula to my back and walk us up to her four-stone sagebrush spot. The cord. Her cord. Our cord.

We squat down and bless it.

"Do you want to dance with your mama?" I ask her blue eyes.

She nods.

I pick her up under her arms, kiss her face, and we spin, spin, spin around the yellow-white field, spinning and laughing into the light. The outdoor dance becomes part of what we do. Here I make contact with my joy. And every Sunday afternoon, while Eula brushes watercolors onto paper, I make a menu for the week and write it up on the blackboard inside of our back door.

Mon—*Kale and red cabbage tahini salad, salmon, sweet potato fries.*

Tues—*Paprika chicken with rice and peas.*

This act helps me.

I call my oldest friend, of the macadamia nut allergy. As we catch up, I decide to expose part of my shadow, one that only Chris and my parents have witnessed. I've pretended to my friends, without consciously knowing it, that I don't do this. She asks me about my last month or two.

"Well, I basically sneak eat when I'm sad," I laugh.

"But, doesn't everyone do that?" she asks.

"I don't know. Do they?"

"Though I did think you ate broccoli and beets when you were stressed."

"C'mon. Really? I gave that impression. *Jesus*," and we both can't stop laughing.

When we stop, I continue, "Clearly there's a shame situation there. No, I go full-force chocolate, cheese, chocolate again, and when I could do gluten, chocolate pretzels."

"I'm eating a bag of chocolate chips right now," she says.

"Oh my god, I wish we could eat them together."

It's not that I want to go down this road of sameness. It's not that I really want to spend my time eating chocolate chips with her. But, a part of me is revealed, a small sparrow hurled out of the nest. The shame comes not from the actual eating. I don't think it's bad to eat chocolate. If I were slender or small, sneak eating could be a casual mention at a party, ha ha, I ate the entire block of cheese, silly me.

But when a round/fat/curvy woman mentions it, people judge.

Who is *she* to eat *that*?

~

I do and don't want to wean Eula. Milk is beyond food—it's connection. I can't yet know what kind of transition this will be for me. I tell her Mama's milk isn't going to be here much longer but that I have loved, loved, loved giving it to her. She hears me. We talk about love in our hearts. Where is your heart? I ask. "Boom boom," she pounds on her chest, my chest. We're down to one nursing a day—in the morning.

It's early October and it's time to stop.

She calls to me at two o'clock in the morning.

"Mama, Mama." I step down the ladder and go to her.

"Come here, sweets," I say, and scoop her up. "Hug your mama, I'm here."

We stand on the cold concrete floor and moonlight pours in from the windows. I bring her to our twin-bed-standing-in-as-couch on the floor.

"You can touch, but no drinking, let's save it for morning," I request.

She understands and rests her head on my shoulder. I could stay here forever, stroke my daughter, her toes, soft back. A few hours later, she inches up and opens her eyes in the dark. Those eyes. Those eyes stared right at me when she was born. She rests her head on my breast and noses down to smell. Her head nods when she is telling me she knows about our agreement.

We stare at each other.

It's hard for me to restrict like this.

I decide to go *halve-sies*, as Mare says, and let her hold my nipple.

"You can hold . . ." I say, but when I pull my tank top back, she mistakes it for an invitation and dives fast, latches, and then sucks milks out super slowly, as if being slow will make me think she isn't there at all.

I try not to laugh.

I snuggle her close and plan to contend with it later.

~

We decide Chris has to be on call for nights because I cannot bear to hear Eula cry for me and not go to her. She's been sleeping well and through the night for a while—a cool cloth over her parents' heads. The ease of consistent sleep for us reminds me how the early sleep deprivation pushed us both into a severely altered state. It doesn't excuse anything but it does help explain it. But now our girl has hit another growth spurt and her rhythm is off. She also senses the end of the boob. Her papa goes to her. If she doesn't stop crying within ten minutes of his soothing, I dash down our stairs and interrupt the whole effort we carefully organized (and promised I wouldn't interrupt) beforehand. About 80 percent of the time, I'm the irritated rescuer.

To avoid this, I remove myself and sleep in my parents' cabin on the daybed.

Otherwise our sleep plan unravels.

It hurts my body to be in a separate house from Eula, and from Chris. But there is no way I can go to her at night and negotiate again. My body wakes at dawn without an alarm. My daughter and I are programmed to each other.

In the dark, I stumble into clothes, walk out onto the porch, and *there*, right there, a lunar eclipse beams at me. There goes the light. Welcome to the shadow. It isn't so bad. I want to lie on the grass and gaze up. I want to place my small self in the galaxy. But tree shadows scare me. Instead, I go to my car and watch it from the safety of my back pressed against a large steel machine.

No one is awake at my home.

I sneak in and lie on the couch—waiting.

"Mama," she calls out.

We venture out together to the cool moon night and her hand digs down my shirt.

"There's the moon," I say.

She freezes, stares. Oh my, Mama. I want her to know cycles and tides and how to trust the moon's bright gaze. We stand cheek to cheek, warm, smell of her lamb's breath, us pressed together, and I think one day I will tell her about this moment.

"So many stars, sweets. See? Sometimes stars shoot out of the sky. You have to watch for them. They are little blessings. They're called shooting stars."

She nods.

We go back to the couch and nurse for an hour.

When she is done, she squirms her naked body up to my face and says, with her finger in the air, "Ta, ta, ta, ta." I try to understand my daughter. What is she saying? Such insistence. Mama, hear me.

"Oh, *star*," I say, "yes, stars, star, star."

Her face relaxes with a nod. She has been understood.

We have a body full of stars.

~

What I learn: Just as women's arousal starts on edges—toes, not sex organs—and moves inward, feminine awareness must descend down-ward into the dark loam before it can ascend. Dark and light coexist. Inconsistency is how we are made. We are *of* the moon, and the moon does not present one way all the time. We are equal to men. We were never meant to be the same. Let's not dilute ourselves to sameness. We women are cyclical. This is about a new feminism.

Some say we must re-wild ourselves.

Go back to blood.

Our anatomy has the most exquisite purpose. Our menstrual cy-cles give us the chance to attune every month. The female body was and is a natural healing and planning system. In the one to two weeks pre-ovulation, a woman has incredible energy for action and doing and projects. When she ovulates, her egg floats and she becomes ripe, alive, sensual, sexual, full, magnetic, a creator matrix awake to her sense and radiance. As she moves into pre-menstruation, the world sharpens. Her laser beam focuses. She becomes a master discerner. She deepens into her intuitive place with a clear, no-bullshit honesty. With that come the uncomfortable moments of magnified feelings. This isn't a place to act from, but a place to gather information. When her blood comes, a woman slows. She goes internal and can connect with the unknown and unseen world. She can let go of the grief from the last month of her life and forgive. Then she pauses at the still point of transition and it starts all over again.

Our hormones guide the cycle.

Our moon waxes and wanes in tandem with the cycle.

My cycle is my teacher.

I have known this for years but my signals got crossed. I've been so devoted to a no-holds-barred expression as part of my right and need as a woman that the idea of timing never occurred to me. If someone told me to save it for later, I would have told that person to stop being the oppressive patriarchy. All along, there was my cycle—*Come back to me, Molly, come back to me, move with me, trust me.* Here is my latest consideration. I've usually said whatever I want in whatever tone I want whenever I want to with Chris. What if, during pre-menses, I did this instead: journal, stomp, pound, cry, scream, but privately, move it through my body alone. Then process those feelings more during menstruation and then, afterward, bring them to him with care. Revolutionary. Better result for everyone. Requires patience.

That is new for me. That is growth.

That is body literacy.

~

As I wean Eula, freshwater lakes enter my dreams. I hope this means something about my own internal lake, my ability to hold my bladder. She woke up with a new word the other day: *baby.* Maybe because you feel like you aren't a baby anymore, sweets.

One morning, loss creeps toward me as I consider the importance of today. I wake early in the cabin, where I have still been sleeping, and walk out into the dark-ink dawn. Once home, I will nurse my daughter for the last time and leave for a book festival—two days of absence, my first absence from her, to seal the deal.

We have timed it well.

As I pad across the lawn toward my car, I stay lost in these thoughts until I lift my head and see a shadow with four legs on the driveway.

What is Bru doing up here so early? Why would he? It couldn't be. Sudden. My body flush, held breath, heart drum, hot scalp let me know it's not him. I backpedal to the guesthouse and slip inside. Now what? No phone. Stranded. There is a mountain lion in the driveway and I need to get home. I open the door and a metallic earth smell hits me. The creek rushes and gurgles. My eyes see shapes that weren't there before. I lean out and say, "Heyyyyyyy-o," and then decide to chance it. Rationally, I know a wild animal wants nothing to do with me. She's probably watching from the trees, waiting for me to leave, so she can continue her night journey. I take a step toward my car, toward where the shadow was. As I make my way, I might be chanting, "It's okay, it's okay," until my hand yanks the driver door open and I catapult my body into safety. In my six years of living here, I have never seen a lion. Blessed by a lion. I drive without headlights and watch for her. When I enter our bright house, Eula toddles up to me, wraps her arms around my calf. I tell them in a flurry, my hands wave all over the place. For the first time, she doesn't ask for milk but I bring her to my breast anyway, try to lock in memory the feeling of her lips on my nipple. Cuddle her up.

We pack my bags into the gray hatchback.

"I'll see you in *two* days," I say to Eula, and I make sure our eyes understand one another. Two days. I love you the most. I love every part of you. When my car turns onto the highway, I am both fractured again and released.

~

People have warned me about the hormonal plummet. When you wean, you can descend for a week or so. "Blues like none other," one of my mama friends described. I have seen some blue so this will only be one more transition for me.

It's easy to forget what you've been told.

Nursing ended a few days ago. So far so good, except that I brought up my sadness about not being seen for my body challenges again and Chris came back at me with the same context argument. I thought I was over it. Guess not.

He falls into a flour-sack sleep after that. Next to him, I stay awake and stare at nothing, me an owl in the middle of the night, watching, waiting, alert.

Body hot.

Body full of fumes.

I sneak down the ladder. Our house becomes a museum: concrete floors, spare wooden furniture, white walls everywhere, dark beyond the windows, windows, so many damn windows. My body leads me to the bathroom. I yank five of my pee-soaked pads out of the trash. I'll show him. With black Sharpie, I scrawl *You don't pay attention* across them. I will hang them on the wall, an artwork, a blaze. They will appear and rock the boat and rock me into recognition. Where is the masking tape? I end up covered in reams of sticky scotch tape, stuck to my pants, my arms. Cannot find any nails, or a hammer. Shit. I line the pads up on the kitchen table instead. He'll see them when he wakes up and when I'm gone. Not sure to where, but I'm out of here.

Except that I'm not.

I can't leave Eula.

That's right, I am a mother of a toddler.

For a few hours, I pace around like a caged animal.

What to do, what to do, what to do?

Then some grace washes over me. Stops me in my tracks. I realize the mistake I'm making. Not now, not in this pre-menstrual-stage weaning moment, not the time for anger at him. Save it for later. Trust your cycle. Open the front door. Release it back to nature. I step onto cold grass, crouch into a ball, and silent scream into my knees for hours. My body moves back inside, where I remove the pads and throw them back in the trash. Crawl up the ladder. Wake Chris up.

"Hold me down, please," I whisper.

"What do you mean?" he asks.

"Put your body on top of mine and don't let me go anywhere."

He does.

I welcome the lead of him.

But he doesn't know what to do with me for the rest of the weekend. He watches from a safe distance and never approaches. I become more and more isolated. In my dream, a brown bear claws at my throat because everyone but me made it to the safety of the forest bathroom. When Eula naps or goes to bed, I collapse on our twin-bed-mattress couch with my face toward the wall and weep. My shoulders hurt from all the heaves.

On Sunday morning, I wake up.

"Let's go get a pumpkin, sweet love," I say to Eula, and button her sweater. We meet Holcomb and her daughter. I don't tell her exactly what I've just done because I don't want to be another downer.

We ride a hay wagon and the girls scream *Woooooo*.

When Eula trips over matted grass, she says, "Boom-ba, Mama," and grins.

When we lounge among the orange globes, surrounded by the spirit of dark and light, I hand Eula seaweed and cranberries and we all laugh and laugh.

~

Slowly, my despair lifts. Who was that woman drawing with Sharpie on her pee-soaked pads? What was she doing?

"Yoo, yoo," Eula says in an attempt to say her own name, "Eula, Eula." We put on music—she likes Michael Jackson or Spanish flamenco the best—and bop around the house, pump our fists in the air. Sometimes, we stir soup or rice and I groove with her on my hip. Sometimes I hold my bladder. Sometimes I don't. I want her close to me, even more now that we don't nurse and because I've been away at student readings for the last few nights.

All I want to do is come home, snuggle up.

I hate being away from her.

There are other songs.

When she hears the mountain song combo from an Argentinean guitar player and Austrian yodeler, she runs from anywhere in the house to leap into my arms. We clutch each other. I spin her and we move across the floor, into the bathroom, her bedroom, spin in the kitchen, flip down, flip up. Mama yodels with the song and then Eula slips her legs on my shoulders, leans back with her chest open to the sky, and we spin.

I want to make a marmalade of this moment.

Preserve it. Put it in the cupboard for when I'm old.

This afternoon, as we dance to a slow Southern song, sway, sway gently, she falls asleep on my shoulder and I don't care if it ruins her nap. Stay there, sweet love. Stay with me.

~

My breasts are honored now, more than ever. One day, Eula stands on our wooden kitchen counter, the same place we chop vegetables together. Autumn sun spreads over us. She pulls open my shirt and touches my bra. I understand she means, *Take them out, Mama*, and I do. She nuzzles her warm face into my chest. Then she cradles one breast in her small hands, hugs and kisses it as if it were a baby bunny. She reaches for the other one and does the same. We are female. We are female love on female. We are adoration of the divine feminine.

She is helping me feel what I want to feel.

"Oh, sweets," I say, and hold her to me.

We gaze out the window and decide to walk to the top of our hill.

It might be our last sunny November day before snowfall.

Sun pokes through a gray sky. The ground spreads golden for miles and miles, that straw color of youth. We lie down on the hump of our hill. Eula crawls over me and flops and flops as our Bru-dog hangs his black jowls over both of us. Sun warms into every cell of us. The whole moment could be a commercial, and what flashes before me are futures—our futures, of growth and who she will be as a girl, and then woman, *how* she becomes herself. When I returned from her eighteen-month doctor visit, my mom asked about it so I gave her the numbers: 37 percent in height. "Oh," my mother had said, as if it were a bad thing. "Well, she just might be short." I had taken a breath and said, *"Moommmm,* who cares? She will be what she will be."

The body is a continued conversation between the women of our lineage.

Remade, like clay.

After Eula's bath, we talk through the day and unscrew the small mason jar of coconut oil. She knows the drill—time to oil her up, a gentle self-care I want her to know about, but not before some crazy naked running around in laps. When she returns, she digs her hand into the jar and comes up with a chunk of fast-melting oil. Slap onto her belly. I rub her arms and back and then she reaches down between her legs.

"Yoo, vulva," she says, and stares up at me.

"Yeah, that's your vulva," I repeat, and try to downplay my sheer exuberance at hearing my daughter say *vulva*, claim *vulva*, for the first time.

~

A few weeks after we wean, I feel changed.

I make an announcement. For the first time in almost two and a half years, since we conceived Eula, I am *me* again. The shadow dark is also me, but here is the everyday me, the woman who doesn't need to explode at someone every other day. I don't want to associate the end of nursing with this feeling, but it's undeniable.

The hormonal shift has affected even my incontinence.

I start going to town with no pads when I'm pre-ovulatory.

I start to brave the world with just underwear under my pants.

Where fallen rocks once covered the tunnel, there is now an open passageway. Life becomes exponentially easier when I'm not peeing on myself. After a sleepless night, I no longer emerge from bed aggravated but eager to put on pad-less underwear. I can snug Eula up in winter clothes, drive to town, buy groceries at three different stores, return home, lug her and them into the house, and not feel destroyed by the end of it. To be almost in control of my bladder restores some ease and a dignity I didn't fully know I'd lost. Instead of energy rushing out of me, it rushes back in.

I start to see glimpses of a healed me. She is real. She moves with grace in the forest, on our plateau, down by the creek. She has let her hair down. That's interesting. When I call out to her, she slips through the trees like a fairy, visible but hidden, moving, never still. Sometimes a gray cloud overtakes her, but she dances with it, sharp movements, kneads it like putty. Sometimes it's a flood of lava or a loud swarm of insects. Same response. She never turns her back. She welcomes. She engages. She moves onward. She shows herself to me.

I am your future, but I am also your past and your present.

What if, instead of the pressure of healing, I just told my body we had a lot of fun exploring ahead of us? Time starts to accelerate. The word *possible* becomes part of my vocabulary again.

"I haven't been capable for so long," I say to Chris.

"*Yes*, you have, you just haven't felt capable," he responds.

"Now I feel glimmers of it."

Capable me.

As She Grew into a Woman

The cosmos set me up—placed me at another college surrounded by gentle green hills and brought full women to my door. These new friends were unlike anyone I had encountered. One woman stood in my dorm room, fresh and pink from a run. The easy way her body moved stunned me. Look at her raise her hands up to reveal prickly armpits. I shaved mine every day. I thought that's what you were supposed to do. Another had done *everything*, drugs, sex, but she didn't brag, she just stated it like, of course, it's fine, whatever. When we sat on the lawn together, she stroked her own leg with reverence. Another held my hand. Often. She would grab and pull me close when something beautiful overcame her—the speckled tree, people singing, something about death she'd read. I went with it, but always questioned why she would want to touch me, of all people.

"You are so beautiful," she would tell me as if it was obvious. Somehow she wasn't measuring my body. She was the first person to tell me about my beauty in a way I could hear.

These women pulled me up from a deep well.

There I was. Within weeks, my self-imposed restrictions began to fall from me like scales. We ran through the woods. We spooned in bed and talked about who we wanted to be. We swam naked. We hung our menstrual cotton pads up in the bathroom. Our senior year we would choose to live in a house together on Cider Mill Road because we wanted to be adult women who lived off campus on a dusty road with such a romantic name. We wanted realness.

The *we* grew me up—to be part of a womanhood I had never seen. They gave me a model.

They gave me a sense of what body aware could be.

They were all slender. I was the largest one, largest breasts, largest hips, largest legs. Somehow (and how it could have been still awes me), these women had no cause for body comparison with me, or each other, and I didn't with them. Without the constant drain of body focus, I was freed. I stepped onto a street whose name I had never really known. The world popped into colors I hadn't seen since girlhood. There was so much to do, so much to be, so much to love.

Six months later, during this sophomore year, at twenty years old, I met Chris. He sat next to me in a writing workshop and, when he spoke, his words were few but profound. What I noticed: long black eyelashes, red down jacket, full-body kindness, scribbles throughout his notebook, schoolteacher parents, born and raised in the mountains of Maine, and he had an ease about him, non-threatening, thoughtful when he told me he liked the scarf in my hair.

I had never pursued a man before.

It took nothing for me to start stalking Chris. I showed up where I knew he would be. I found him across campus, down dorm halls, on the dining patio. After patting my own cheeks in the mirror and saying, *Do it*, I dialed his four-digit room number from my dorm phone and asked him to go on a hike. He picked me up in his old pale blue hatchback and gave me an orange. We lumbered through an icy winter forest and spoke of moose. I didn't know what kind of tracks were in the snow. "Maybe you don't know this animal?" he asked. We were islands reaching out to each other. I was led by a bravery beyond me. I would have never done what I did if some other force hadn't been guiding me. Cut to the chase. I sat next to him on my bed and told him dead-on, "I like you." He reciprocated. He wrote poems for me. He drew shape-shifter animals and slipped them under my door.

We had sex for the first time on Good Friday.

In my room, and other rooms, we would unravel each other for the rest of college, slowly, faster, under the moon, layers and layers of my sadness peeled away, as we found words and nonwords, as we learned what it meant to be a body in love. It was easy, somehow, for me to undo the clench of my legs with him.

"You've been through so much," he would say, and I would deflect his empathy and correct him and say, No, not really, not at all, besides, one in four women have been violated by a man. He'd gone to a large public school where many of his peers struggled with drugs and abuse. He was aware. But he didn't have sisters. Maybe the complex world of women was new to him.

He seemed so innocent to me.

I was innocent too.

We used three types of birth control at the start, until a friend pulled me aside and said, "It's not necessary, you know?" You mean it isn't normal to be on the pill and have him wear a condom and shoot spermicide inside your vagina? I was not going to get pregnant. Despite my diligent pee-after regime, I got recurrent urinary tract infections. "What does a UTI feel like?" he asked. Like someone is sticking an uncooked fettuccini noodle up my urethra. It evolved into a sort of cystitis. A doctor gave me an antibiotic to take every time we had sex for a month. Let's say approximately fifty-six pills in four weeks for young-love sex frequency. No mention of probiotics. I didn't know. The urinary tract infections went away and I remained unaware of the link between bladder and unresolved anger. Whatever anger I held had nothing to do with him anyway.

He was a gentle shepherd.

He couldn't stop touching my back, my strong tan back.

Each time he asked me to please please please stand naked and face away from him, I couldn't do it. I couldn't show my butt with sunshine coming into the window. He didn't understand. I heard myself say the same thing about my butt my mother had said about her butt even though we didn't really have the same butt.

Orgasms were an effort for me.

I never felt unsafe with him, but unsafe with my own let go. I would barely let him explore. Many of my women friends, even those I would have never suspected, had a similar issue—how was this possible? One friend and I bought three books about the female orgasm.

Chris watched me read them and weep. "It'll be okay," he said, kissed my forehead, and then told me he would do anything I needed him to do. It wasn't that. I couldn't explain that it had nothing to do with him. Something much larger than us had shut down my capacity to relax and feel; something beyond my violation in Paris; something layered in how we talked about women, how women were trained to feel about their bodies, how women believed they should give, not receive. When my mother saw the books tumble down from my closet a few years later, she said, "Eww," and leapt away as if they were toxic. I steeled myself and spat, "They aren't my books, anyway."

On my last day of college, I shaved my head.

That night, Chris rubbed my fuzzy skull. How did it look? Different, was all he could say. We were parting ways after college. Not a breakup, but I had insisted we needed to date other people so we could really choose each other. "But, we're in love," he had protested. I told him it didn't matter, we had to do it, and so he agreed. He was headed to an island in the South Seas to study geology, and my future lay in the red rock desert. We stroked each other, wrapped up in what felt like the end of youth.

I told him I wanted to learn about natural medicine.

"You *should*, babe, you'd be great at that," he said, and we touched noses.

"But I don't have anything wrong with my body," I said, eyes up at the ceiling, awake with life. "And I want to test it on me, I want to have my own experience with herbs, all of it."

Later, he would remind me of what I had called to me.

I moved to New Mexico to work with girls at a boarding school.

That year electrocuted me.

On my first evening among adobe and blue sky, I ended up in the ER with a racing heart rate and strange disorientation. The doctors gave me applesauce. There was nothing physically wrong. The school campus, surrounded by ponderosa pines, smelled of vanilla and dry and West. This lit me up. Made me feel wild. The men I worked with seemed drawn to me, my freedom, detachment, strong legs, the way I took off into the woods alone, the way I didn't care about my short strange grown-out hair. Being the desired one made me feel more desirable. I began to understand that putting attention on dress didn't need to be a superficial act done for others. I had always assumed it to be so. I could self-decorate. I could call my body a landscape to honor with jewelry and colors. It wasn't bad to wear mascara or choose the blue scarf to match my eyes or take more than five minutes to decide upon a pair of pants that actually fit.

There was a man: blond, former cocaine addict, motorcycle, and literature. On a school adventure, we counselors slept in sleeping bags around a campfire and he and I found each other. Afterward he said, "Now I know what glowworm sex feels like," even though we hadn't had penetrating sex. I was guarded with him. We giggled and then I got up in the dark to puke in a clump of sagebrush. He had known hundreds of women. His body was not safe to me.

But he opened a deep uncontrolled part of me.

I met a woman who became my ally. On weekends, we walked across mesas at dusk and rode through arroyos on her tandem bicycle. She showed me how to chart my menstrual cycle. Gone with the birth control pill. Our gorgeous red blood! My cycle. What an honor to have my own cycle to connect me to other women, women now, women of the past, to the moon. I learned that egg-white stretchy cervical fluid means fertile. I learned to feel for the way my cervix hardened and softened to a peach during a month. My body temperatures were low and the books indicated it might be a sign of thyroid imbalance. I didn't know what a thyroid was. Though a vibrator had helped me like it does many women, I packed it away and explored with only my hands, found breath and a natural pace that invited me into my primal self. When my friend practiced her cranial sacral therapy on me, she would say, "Oh, Molly, you are *wide* open."

I was finally awake to myself.

But with such opening came that disorientation and spinning, a spinning so brutal I often cried out to a god, to someone, anyone. I would rather die than experience the flutter in my heart as it crawled up my throat every single night. Sometimes I sat on the gravel road and used a phone card to call Chris across the ocean. He didn't know what to say about the spinning. I would ask him to stay on the phone with me anyway. He would. He was often silent, so I was too. We were both too stunned. My parents suggested it might be panic attacks—but I had no use for modern medicine diagnoses, or for my parents those days. When my mother had seen my fertility-awareness chart on my nightstand, she picked it up and started to read—creamy, egg-white—and then tossed it away with an "Oh, uh, gross." Really, Mom? If I had panic in me, something else lay beneath and I would unearth it. When the spinning consumed me, I crawled out of my white trailer into the moonlight where I could find a juniper to clutch. The ghost smell of juniper and pinion would turn me on or turn me off.

Me, in my underwear, as the scratch bark scratched me back to my senses.

I couldn't see it was a portal opening, the start of my feminine wanting to wake up at my root, to spin me open. I wasn't ready for it then. Too much fear of what would awaken, of what it was.

Strange things happened to my body. I saw a healer who wore only gray sweats and ate only raw meat. From a sample of my blood, he could read my history, down to the actual events, down to violation. He cleared them for me. Was that possible? I found flecks of black in my urine. When my menstrual blood turned to sludge, he nodded, "Good." Clear it all out. In a dress shop, a woman with cat-eye sunglasses told me a worm had lodged in my brain from drinking bad water in the woods (I had spent the summer in the woods) and that I was sleeping with someone dirty (my new dangerous man friend). Everyone now had an opinion. She continued to click her words at me until I said *Stop* and walked out. I learned to stand on my head and to weep in savasana. My dreams of shit and blood came through every night now—so much of it.

My parents came to visit. We walked through the Santa Fe plaza where my mother had dropped me off and cried a year earlier. I could now sense her doing something behind me. I turned to find her coming at the back of my head in public with her Mason Pearson brush, trying to brush my unruly short hair down.

"God, Mom," I yelled, and walked further and then farther away.

A few weeks later, my coworker's car spun out on ice and we rolled in just the way I had foreseen we would. My houseplants leapt from shattering terra-cotta pots and soil sifted down over upside-down us. One well-placed rock prevented us from plummeting into the river. Then a naturopath gave me a liver tonic. She told me my liver wasn't functioning at 100 percent, which I heard as my liver wasn't functioning. A psychic told me three things: I had been born under a dark moon, my life-partner man would work with his hands, and my only path to salvation was through expression.

None of this helped my night attacks.

I chose to believe my wounds and strange experiences made me special, deep.

My departure from the red rock desert coincided with the disappearance of my night attacks, or a new pathway for them. I moved to New Zealand to work on farms, learn about food systems, and be near my love. Chris had picked me up at the small airport in the red 1964 Volkswagen bug he fixed up. The ether smelled sweet here, an island so near the island of my birth. After more than a year apart, after a year of another lover for each of us, our hands fit with a new sort of grip. He continued his study of geology and I drove to a valley four hours away. I pulled on canvas work pants, bumped up a dirt road to a farmhouse, and asked a barrel-chested man for a job.

He stared me up and down.

He let me feel the pause.

"Most women prefer the packing house," he said, referring to standing over a conveyer belt in a loud warehouse to sort the good fruit from the bad.

"I would rather work outside," I stated.

"Okay then," he said, and the grin on his face foretold his approval of what he would later call my grit. I would get paid for how much I picked and share a bunkhouse with other workers from the Czech Republic, China, Malaysia, and Sweden.

The apple trees smelled of wax. The work was hard—apples heavy on a reversed backpack, eight-hour nonstop days, and metal ladders hot under a sun and thin ozone layer. Tree climber. My young self would have wanted nothing more. In the shower, I watched dirt wash from my tan, slender, strong body. This efficient body was the body I was meant to live in. My friends and I were now in our mid-twenties.

Those back in the States somersaulted toward advanced degrees and professions. But all I wanted to do was move my body.

I stayed on for pear and cherry and apricot seasons.

I was the only woman and the fastest picker of the bunch—always comfortable as the leader in a group of men who were as tame as younger brothers. One afternoon, I drove them to a lake across the river to shuck off our heat. My normal reservations about being seen in a green bikini or any swimsuit didn't apply here in a mix of cultures and ages and stages.

One man from India poked my stomach.

"I didn't expect this from you," he said. I couldn't believe he had said so and just gone ahead and touched my woman belly softness. He caught me off guard. I had a flat stomach. Did he expect a six-pack? He wasn't trying to offend. It surprised him because of the way I ran around the orchard.

"I guess I didn't expect it from myself either," I said.

"Okay," we both laughed. No one had ever made a comment about my body in such non-judgmental plain-speak.

When each season ended, as the wet winter approached, I returned to Chris with the scent of flowers and boxes of fruit in my car. Some part of me aware of how a goddess could awaken in me.

"You are a new woman," he would say, and grab for me in his breezy flat.

For work in his town, I modeled nude for an art class. Somehow I had no qualms about taking my robe off. The only hard part was sitting still. The scent from a nearby chocolate factory wafted in through old, creaky, lead-paint windows. The teacher turned on guitar music, and they all drew me as a version of themselves. It became an evening of adoring the female form. During the break, they invited me over to their canvases to show me how wonderful it had been to draw this line or that curve.

I was becoming a beautiful woman.

Part of my dam had crumbled, but my "new me" collapsed with anxiety when I was quiet or still, and I reverted around family. Lauren came to visit me with her best friend. The three of us traveled around the island, camping on rock beaches and in ditches and fields. They stood out. Blond. Tan. Confident. When they strut into gas stations, all eyes would turn.

Somewhere, in a corner, was me, a shadow no one could see.

In their presence, I allowed myself to become less than I actually was.

I hid my sorrow about it by being the leader, again. I drove the car, and once they both told me my hands were lovely. But it seemed a token.

My hands.

My hands.

Yet working with my hands helped me touch my beauty. I vowed to ask a future daughter one day—how do *you* feel gorgeous, radiant, feminine, what ways or moments draw that up in you?

For me, it was body movement. I knew that now. As long as I could move, I could embody beauty. Pull me up a tree. Haul that heavy box. Do a cartwheel. Though my mother had modeled this way for me in her own container of life, for her it was out of necessity, less out of her personal desire. Had any of my ancestors felt body connected to earth? On a seaweed farm, after dragging long dark green strands of kelp from sand beach to garden, I stood at the edge of a wild ocean and understood all my woman ancestors had indeed been of the earth. Every one descends from people who have worked land and depended on nature.

Two years later, when our plane coasted back across the equator, I landed in Boston and went back to the land: drove tractors, carried boxes of heavy vegetables, worked with teens again, and swam in ponds.

It wouldn't be my endgame.

I knew so.

But my grounded female had found a home with the earth. It was a natural posture for me. I began to dream of ground animals—rabbits, mice, marmots—holding out small pills of medicine for me in their tiny paws.

My mother was glad to have me back in the country.

One afternoon, she sat on my bed and watched me undress from work.

"This life suits you, Moll," she said, and gazed at me. She meant my slenderness must be an indication of my happiness. I didn't call her on it. However she saw it, I knew she could also see the pleasure of my body in nature, in labor.

Shed

Eula teaches me every moment can be a prayer. She is sick. Her sinus, ears, nose, throat are working it out. We are not home. We are in Texas visiting a friend. We sleep in the backyard guesthouse cradled by humid fragrant air. Neighborhood cats prowl and scream outside. I strip her down naked. Must remind myself that, though her mama runs cold, she runs hot. We move around in the unfamiliar bed, brick-red sheets, awake, awake, awake. My face presses against her soft warm back as she snuggles closer. I wrap my arms around her small torso and she grabs my thumbs. Together, our hands make hands in prayer. Trees rustle and shadows dance over us. I will be with you wherever you are, whatever new beds you sleep in, wherever in the world as you grow, even when you don't want me, here I am, my arms around you.

Twenty minutes later, Eula moves around for a new position.

We thrash together until birds sing their song.

~

When we return, my prayers accumulate—thank you. Weaning has freed me. Please let me make use of this new field of flowers before me. I have been a horse frothing at a closed starting gate. The gate has opened. My legs stretch long and there is somewhere to go, somewhere un-trapped.

Then, one day, my mom's car crashes. I'm driving home from client meetings, planning how to get Eula more fabric for her folding obsession, when I get a text: *Upside down in a ditch off Enders. Am okay.*

I keep going on the snowy road because I'm almost to Enders. *On my way,* I text back and assume her car careened in one of the two-foot ditches so common out here. We'll need some chains. We might have to call a tow company. But then I can't find her. I can't find her anywhere.

Where are you? I text.

Then I see her head as she climbs out of a twenty-foot ditch.

Jesus.

I get out of my car and run across the empty country road. When I hug her, electricity surges from her skin. Are you okay? Are you okay? She is unhurt. Her eyes flash alive, angel-like. We peer over the edge at her smashed car. I don't understand how she is okay. If she had been knocked out, we wouldn't have found her. If this had happened in deep winter, under snow, we wouldn't have found her. I didn't even know this ditch was there.

"Let's get you warm," I say as we make our way to my car. She explains that she slid on the ice, and then *woop*, there went the car. By the time we leave, she's made friends with the policeman and tow guy. I keep insisting that we have someone check out her neck, but she tells me she's fine.

I spend that night with her in the cabin. My father is in New York and I want to be sure she's okay, even though nothing on her body hurts.

"I don't want you to elbow me if I snore," she says, so I sleep on the daybed.

When we wake, we sit around in our blue-and-white Japanese bathrobes (*yukatas* leftover from her parents' sojourn there) and drink tea.

"You don't hurt at all, Mom?"

"Not at all. I feel *alive*," she says.

"I can't believe your mom wasn't hurt," Chris says. Even he is moved to an exclamation. My mother rarely feels physical pain, even when a branch gouged her leg bloody, when she cut a sliver of her finger off chopping vegetables, when she had shoulder surgery, when she burned her hand with oil, when her "bulge" was protruding from her vagina. Maybe my long-term interest in the body has made that sort of detachment not an option. I have a different trajectory. That's okay.

~

In her bright office, Holcomb does internal pelvic work on me, part of her training. I lie covered on a table and she massages the vaginal tissue to release holding. It doesn't alarm me to have her fingers inside me.

"It's a wonder," she says, "we have standard bodywork on all other parts of the body except this one." Every woman holds her female history in the pelvis. We watch the way our mothers and grandmothers walk. We watch what they protect and what they leave vulnerable. We take note of whether they dance, and how they dance. Because we are programmed to mimic, we do. But beyond observance, we have genes. They turn on or off based on what circumstances life sends our way.

What might live between my hips? The inherited belief systems are hard to identify. They can feel so far from my own but they have spawned my own. I have spent so much of my life trying to shed them. But there are others I've not recognized. Years ago, a massage therapist had encouraged me to meditate on my pelvic bowl. I had visions of spending a weekend drawing the ligaments, making the hammock shape out of clay, wearing all red during the process, meditating on my pelvis every full moon. It never happened. There was never a large-enough cause to spearhead the action.

Holcomb rouses me from wherever I've been on her table in a dark room. She lets me come to and then shares what she noticed: gentle tone, no significant prolapse, stagnation, scar tissue from the surgery, upper right quadrant slow to respond, left side bound, and lots of heat. It's a lot to receive, but she says it in a way that normalizes it.

"You can do this work on yourself," she shares.

I walk into the January winter aware of my holding, eager to release it.

~

What I learn: My incontinence has woken me up to rage, and rage has woken me up to the remarkable Mama Earth voice in my pelvis. It has been locked up—for eons. It is specific to my life and also unspecific, ancestral, beyond me but in me. It isn't bad. I'm not meant to banish it from my essence (you can't do that anyway). It is a teacher, an energy to sculpt, transmute, and, here's the most important step, direct with care and intention.

Amass the uterine lining.

Release the egg.

Float the egg.

Shed the lining.

Ground yourself after blood.

Rage might be part of my medicine. It has been both my destroyer and my healer.

~

Healing really *does* happen for people. Maybe these people are more practical. Perhaps they have not constructed a worldview that a wound never shakes free from the body because it has become part of your important human story—or even an ally. Now I'd rather have no story and the ability to trapeze and cartwheel. I wouldn't have dared or wanted to make that trade two years ago.

Eula is approaching her second birthday. When she falls, she smooches her own knee. At first, this awes me. How does she know? But then I remember I taught her to do that and must remind myself of my own self-care. She wants to tend to everyone's *Boom-bas*, investigate and track the progress of Papa's blister, Mama's stubbed toe, Mare's finger cut. If I've had a cold, she strokes my throat and asks, "Your throat better, Mama?" I choose to believe this interest is developmental or a part of her inherent curiosity, not a response to having witnessed a wounded mother.

By nature, she wants to soothe.

She hugs the animals in her books, leans her face onto the page and snuggles them as best you can snuggle a hard-edged story. On one page, two children bury a dead chipmunk as butterflies surrounded them. I understand this metaphor for death, but she furrows her brow and stares up at me, "Awwww, okay?"

"Well, that chipmunk died," I explain. "She's going back to the earth. It's okay, everything dies, sweets, we all die, it's a natural process." I refuse to make up a lie. I know she won't absorb what I'm saying completely, but she also *knows*. She just came from that place. She knows even as she tries to sort it out in her mind.

"There you go," she says, and strokes the chipmunk, "there you go."

When I hear my own language coming from my daughter's mouth, I hear the frequency of my *There you go*. We flip the page to a scene of turtles, deer, and storks resting by a stream. She steps her feet on the page and inches closer, trying to push her way into that world. Her green-striped socks slip. She wants to go there. I get it. Determined, she turns her whole body around and tries to back in with her bum. Maybe that's the key. Then she attempts with her arms shot out. No luck.

I've been watching her transport herself these days. She and Mare have a ritual of doing "lipstick." One afternoon, I made dinner in the kitchen and watched her. She picked an orange crayon from her art box and flopped down on our low couch. After a contented sigh, she stared up at the ceiling and began to paint her whole mouth orange, over and over again, for an hour, no pause.

Where was she?

These private moments multiply.

At bedtime now, she wants to tweak the hell out of my nipple. I usually don't mind, except when the sensation of wanting my body back swoops over me. One evening, I said, "No thank you, Eula, no nipple tonight." When she huffed and puffed and blew my house down, I gave in to my exasperation and barked, "Just go to sleep, just go to sleep, please." I slunk off to bed with the chest ache of having said the wrong thing to my child.

The next night, after my planned glass of white wine and some chocolate, we sit on her blue rug together with the lights off. When she reaches for me, I cup my own breasts and don't move. The look of confused betrayal in her eyes is hard for me to watch. She pounds on my chest, scrapes at me, tries to pry my hands away.

"I know, sweets, I know, I know it's hard," I repeat.

But she rages more, hurls her body on the bed and then pounds on my legs. I breathe and tell her *I'm here, I'm here, I'm here* as she screams. I want to reach out to her but then my breasts become available. Under the dark canopy of her room, I wait for the energy to move through her. Her movements are familiar. We all do this. When her body collapses on me, I hug her to my chest and feel her fury evaporate.

"There you go, Eula, there you go. I'm here."

~

At my yearly women's exam, my second one since Eula's birth, I realize I don't know what exactly caused my incontinence or minor prolapse. I assumed the vacuum, pushing for five hours, the natural posture of my body, but maybe not. Somehow knowing what it was will help me heal.

"I'm looking for a *why*," I ask my gynecologist, the kind one from before.

"It's hereditary," she says. "I've seen women with five kids, or women who push for hours and hours, and you'd never know they had a baby. Some women have a textbook birth and tons of postpartum challenge. It's about connective tissue, and often your mother's pelvic floor is your own. The vacuum and pushing didn't help, but they probably weren't the direct cause."

I'm shocked.

It makes complete sense. It's also her opinion, one opinion. I tend to believe it's all of the above. It's everything. It isn't just one reason. But part of me *is* made this way. What does that mean? Afterward, my gray hatchback cradles me in the parking lot. My body feels liberated and bound at the same time by this information. No event to blame. No person to blame. My inheritance. But I must choose what to do with it.

I go home with a sort of health resolution.

When our house darkens, I sit on a chair in our loft with a towel underneath half of my butt and do a Kegel, as if on a horse. This is one exercise from the pelvic-floor audio CD I recently bought—one to add to my collection of barely used ones. But on this cover, a woman leaps on a beach. I want to leap again. The woman, trained as a Feldenkrais practitioner, healed herself after two births and some significant incontinence. Her story becomes my beacon. I can no longer afford to be inconstant with my pelvic-floor exercises simply because I have been in denial or anger. It is no longer such a shock. I'm beyond that part now.

What if I befriend my bladder and my pelvic bowl?

Give them a name. Talk to them; believe in their capacity to heal, instead of berating them. Tell them we can do this together. When Chris and Eula run races on the driveway, the wrecking ball returns heavy on my chest. I feel separate. I don't want to be separate anymore. In a recent dream, Eula and I both have red-splotched birthmarks. They begin at our thyroids and flame up all over our throats. I ask Chris to rub calamine lotion on us and he does, but we aren't sure whether it'll go away.

When I wake up, the *no* from my body sets a boundary with the great beyond.

Don't you dare make this part of her body story one day.

Don't you dare.

February unfolds more snow and more snow and more snow, as usual. When we drive to town and stop at a light, I hold my bladder and say, *I see you, I honor you, I'm here,* and then Eula, from the back, sees the green light and calls out:

"Green! Go, Mama, go."

~

There is the healing of my body. There is the healing of my relationships.

I wish I could believe they are separate.

That would be convenient, easier.

188

My mom and I are in synch these days. One afternoon, we sort through Eula's clothes—put away the small ones and integrate the hand-me-downs. Sun pours through her bedroom window and Eula stands naked in a drawer on the floor and dresses up.

"I remember getting all her clothes ready before birth. So neat and tidy," I laugh.

"Yeah, you can't know what's coming, can you?" my mom says.

We re-story, day by day. I could never let my mother love me by offering clothes because I couldn't love myself. Clothes have now, for the most part, become a connection point. I have chosen to make it so. My mother leaves tomorrow to visit my brother in Thailand. I don't want this domestic moment of ours to end. I already miss her.

"What do you think about these pants?" I ask.

"Pitch 'em."

"These?"

"Those will last another few months."

During the three weeks she is gone, I clean the guesthouse for the rental guests. My mother is present everywhere—the way she folds rags, leaves a pad of butter out for cooking, stores her grains in a basket, keeps her spiritual books on a cherry wood table by her bed. Her absence is a hole in my stomach. It's acute. And I come to understand how necessary her being here has been for me. She has been the familiar background—the person Eula and I can walk down the dirt driveway to see, the one who knows how long the salmon should be in the oven, the mother who says, "It's okay. You just can't go there right now." It makes sense to navigate motherhood with your mother.

I would have been very isolated without her.

She filled in when Chris was unavailable.

Maybe this is how it has always been: the women together, the men in and out.

Now that we live in our house, he has gathered some of his energy back—works normal hours on furniture, comes in for dinner with us and we all say thank you to the great elk spirit, leans close to me as we discuss what kind of couches he might build for us one day. We thread our partnership back together and touch our pain as we do so.

Bloodletting.

Woozy.

We are acting out a gender dance, a systemic healing of what men have done to women and women have done to men, part ours but also older than us. It's been a mutual violence. Men have wronged men too. What would this process be if my lover were a woman? Women have wronged women too. The discomfort of our growing encourages me out of the house. I am holding on to the lifeboat that reminds me one person cannot nor should meet all my needs. I am trying to change my tendency to rarely reach out to friends when in need. I meet one in a restaurant. At midnight, I drive to one's house with puffy eyes and tears streaming. With another, I walk. They all understand the nuance of my marriage without me saying much because somehow it is the nuance of their marriages too. We do not live in cocoons. Exhaustion can swallow my intentions. What I'm saying is I don't know if I can do it, if I have the strength to heal both my body and my marriage, and they need to happen together.

One friend reminds me about radical self-acceptance.

Another passes on what someone passed to her: You do, he sees. It's on you.

Another friend tells me to throw my diagnosis, not myself, off a cliff.

They are all saying, Assume a posture. One evening, he puts Eula to sleep and I leave on foot with cranberry lip stain in my pocket. We haven't had an argument. We aren't triggered by one another in this moment. I move up the hill behind our home, past owls and hawks above and coyotes somewhere, to engage in my own prevention ritual. I need a red mouth for it. I want a red mouth as part of my body. I have learned about the importance of self-decoration from my daughter. On goes my red mouth and, near trees, on the open flat, mountains watch or don't, as I spin and spin and spin and shake myself down into the earth.

For hours.

When I return, everyone slumbers and, then, so do I.

~

At the end of March, we meet up with some of Eula's friends at a park. Under the linden trees, spring calls to us all, grass, sun, warmth at long last. The dogs run around in a pack, as do our toddlers. Eula breaks from the group and runs far away, down to the bottom meadow. I sit with the other mothers and watch. Thought I'd be done with my healing by now: another spring, another chance for renewal.

She smooches each tree.

Runs with her hands above.

Laughs to herself.

A boy rolls down the hill and his mother follows him, rolling. I take note of the way she hugs to her core. I want so much to do that too but worry my body will break. It is time to step out of what has been. Let wounded woman dissolve back to the earth, or at least let her rest. Soon. Look at my teacher, Eula, and how she runs.

I will mimic my daughter.

~

Eula screams for me before dawn. I scamper down the ladder, walk across the concrete floor, and crouch down by her bed.

"What's wrong, sweets?" I ask.

"Owls get you," she mumbles. "Owls get you." By *you*, she means her. The owls have been hooting outside her window. I grab the down comforter, crawl into her warm bed, and cuddle up with her.

"Hold nipple, hold nipple," she says, and grabs on, her safety always, at the grocery store, in any circumstance she needs comfort. She hands me a stuffed animal; if she has one, I should have one too.

"They won't get you, sweets, they're just saying, *Hello, Eula. Hello, Eula,* when you hear them," I explain as we wrap up, press nose to nose, and fall asleep together.

My dreams come, too.

My dreams will come like a great migration this spring.

I dream of a tattooed woman. She tells me I've passed away. I tell her I haven't. "Yes you have," she says.

We wake up wrapped up in each other, and Eula pushes up, ready for her day. I pretend to be asleep but can sense her blue eyes watching me. It's a good thing to pass away in a dream. Time to enter a passage and leave the old behind. Why is death so much like birth?

~

"Sorry, Mama," Eula says one day when she bumps into me at the front door. I've never heard her say *sorry*, and it bothers me that she says it in this context. No need for that word so overused by women. I bend down and put my arm around her.

"You don't have to say *sorry*, you just say, *excuse me*," I explain. I realize *excuse me* has its own set of issues, but the word *sorry* frightens me. It's the gateway drug to all the other words women use to apologize for their own existence. Clearly I say it often—sorry I was late, sorry I didn't tell you, sorry sorry sorry. In our early days, Chris used to say, "Babe, you don't have to say *sorry* when you tap me on the shoulder to ask me a question."

I need to erase it from my weekly vocabulary.

I want to preserve it for when I really mean it.

Eula nods.

Later that afternoon, Eula runs through the house. Her bare feet tap tap the concrete floor and she sings, "Sorry, sorry, sorry, sorry," as she glances back at me with a grin. Oh, girl. I don't respond but love her defiance, this feedback loop. When I start saying, *excuse me*, she will follow.

~

What I learn: Our language is the language of our dominator culture. It has become familiar; we no longer recognize it. We use it to exert power over another. I want to tend to language. It's my thing. It's the one choice and intention I feel most sure about as a parent. I know I will make mistakes. Everyone calls animals *he* (unless the animal has a baby), so I call almost every animal we see *she*. When winter rolls around again, we are going to build a snowwoman: snowmen too, but a snowwoman first. Why aren't there more snowwomen? I also won't call a poop diaper *dirty* because poop isn't dirty. It's poop. Nothing from our body is dirty. We rewrite "Baa, Baa, Black Sheep" with a queen and little girl who lives down the stream. I know Eula will grow up in a mélange of words and worlds and that is good, but I want to give her a foundational sense, through everyday language, that equal footing between genders should exist.

The pendulum has got to swing for that to happen.

I would have made the exact same word adjustments with a son.

Because it's a myth that only women suffer from the patriarchy.

Men do too.

They get shut down. They benefit from the system on a thick surface level—jobs, power, control—but the expectations for a man to be "a man" can be brutal and unyielding. It might be easier for a girl to be a tomboy than a boy to be, what? Other men expect them to be *men*. Don't lose your manhood. I've never heard of a woman telling a woman not to lose her womanhood, though the subtext of what women expect of each other is equally complicated. I don't mean to understate or overlook that it's been harder for women, but I no longer want to be the person who demeans men in order to find a place for women. There is such unexplored terrain for men. It hasn't been safe for them to access their own feminine essence. Actually, it hasn't been safe for anyone. Women of my generation have been trained to be masculine. Out of need. Out of era. Out of an attempt to match the world's pace. But my own overblown masculine has caused significant pain—to me, to my loved ones. On many levels, I have been the very patriarchy I abhor.

We don't see the feminine anywhere in our culture.

It barely exists in our collective language, actions, or policies. Bless those on the forefront of gender conversation. Gender fluidity is shaking it all up, reminding us that the feminine and masculine energy can coexist in each person, each town, each country.

This isn't about female takeover.

But the shift includes an overdue recognition of the female body.

~

At the base of my throat, an apology has begun to grow. It happens slowly in everyday moments when he, the main *he* in my life, walks past our kitchen table to get a glass of water and touches my shoulder just because, like he used to; when he emerges naked from a shower, strong shoulders and strong butt, and Eula asks about his penis and he doesn't skip a beat, says, "Yep, that's my penis," and continues toweling off his head; when he becomes obsessed with playing the ukulele for Eula as she dozes off; when he leaves uncapped pens around the house, trademark move of his; when he peeks around the corner, runs toward his daughter, swoops her up and tosses her high to then catch her and her giggles; when he teases me about the vocabulary I make up by saying *Only Molly*; when my parents ask him to chainsaw a fallen tree and he gets right to it; when he shares some obscure fact about geology or Syria or the way an airplane works; when he makes his coffee first and Eula's scrambled eggs second and she doesn't goad him like she does me; even when he says in the dark, "We are both triggered, let's leave it until tomorrow"; even when he is tired and hunched and silent and covered in sawdust.

I have begun to see my husband again.

I don't know what part of my lens has been real or not real.

The bud in my throat starts to unfurl. Somehow, now, it might not require an apology from him in order to bloom itself. I have said I'm sorry a thousand times, with half breath, in stolen moments, twice with tears and what I thought was meaning, though usually, not always, with a condition: if I say it, he must say it back to me. His silence, any deliberate silence, can be its own form of violence. I do believe that still.

But enough.

There is an apology.

It is alive and green in me.

It is feral and of my flesh.

It has words but does not want to use words.

How can I communicate this with my body: I'm not sorry for my feelings but I'm sorry it was so messy, for my attacks and demands on you every day, for wanting closeness five minutes later, for that whiplash, that new parenthood wasn't what we expected, that I could not be the glowing new mother and you didn't even require that of me, for all the blame, the way I undervalued your contribution because I wanted mine to be seen, for the unsafe space, and that I hurt you enough so you, tender you, could not be tender with me.

~

I step out of our concrete shower, away from our green plants, and bend down naked to put Eula's books back in a basket. We are cleaning up. She dances around behind me and then goes to crawl through my legs. I glance through my own legs at her paused, face-to-face with my vulva, looking at it with big wide *Oh my goodness* eyes. What is that, what is that place?

I don't say anything.

I watch her take stock.

I will never forget those eyes.

Later that week, Eula stands in the bathroom with me as I change my pad. She sees blood and asks, "Owie, Mama, boom-ba?" As she scuffs her feet on the wood floor, I explain that it's my blood, not a wound. I say the word *period* even though I want to say *menses*. *Menses* seems not part of street language, so I opt out of it. For the next four days, she watches, checks my pad, helps me fold it up and put it in the trash. She asks if she can touch the blood. Yes, you can. Can she smell it? Sure. Eula marvels that a tampon goes in me and comes out. I tell her over and over again this part of being a woman. It's good and not scary. One day she'll have blood too. I wonder what of it she understands.

A few days after my blood is gone, we walk though our small backyard forest: over mossy rocks, under cottonwoods, near the baby woodpecker nest. I try my latest vow to lead with my pelvis. It's not a jut out, more of a sway, more like my eyes reside between my hips. The world smells of water.

Ahead, Eula patters along and chants to herself.

"Mama woman, Mama period. Papa no. Bru no. Mama woman. Eula girl. Eula woman. One day."

~

Chris puts his head between my legs and I light up from the inside. What I need to trust: we are part of coming back to some center. He can sense a change in me too. In the dark, trees stand somewhere beyond our pane of glass. Motherhood has made me more animal than ever before, unbound by what came before me, more in tune with the feminine art of receiving. Remember you were born a sensual person and you will continue to learn well into old womanhood all the ways it is safe to be sensual. Waves start to pass through me. No expecting a man to make me feel this way, not this man, not any man. But when it happens, I accept. I cannot only do physical pelvic exercises and take thyroid medicine.

There is more.

The wilderness within me needs a voice.

My inner current depends on my tending.

As we love-make in the loft, this connection is everything I want right now.

"Mama," Eula screams. Oh no. Oh no. I plead with her telepathically, *Please just an hour, then I will come down.* But it doesn't work and she has a cold, so I pull him up.

"I know," he breathes. "We should go down."

We means *me.*

I go down, smelling of heat, and soothe her, give her my nipple to hold in the dark until she falls asleep again. I climb back up the ladder to the warm body of my husband, his strong hands, and pull his face to mine: my body, his body.

We have spoken decades to one another.

"I wasn't done with you," he says, and then he descends down the length of my body, back down to my root, to me, to the root.

~

Holcomb works on my pelvic bowl again. Her fingers move along the scar tissue. She asks me to signal if it's too much. Lying on the table, I close my eyes to the bright sun and the sensation of an eight out of ten on the pain scale—a hot iron smoothes out the tissue and the burn of it goes deep, beyond, out to far edges of my hip.

I can handle it.

I will handle it if it is meant to help me.

At the end of our session, she swivels on her stool and stares at me. "Your body responds fast," she says. "Faster than most." Many body-workers have told me my body shifts quickly.

Remember that.

Remember how willing my body is.

Remember how my mother has always told me my body heals fast.

"That was super intense, I mean, super intense."

"Yeah," she sighs. "I hope not too much. Remember, this kind of deep work can loosen some feelings too, so be gentle with yourself. I also noticed an energy, almost got knocked off my chair by it. You're holding on to a collective suffering and it isn't serving you."

"That feels so vast," I say, and I start to sit up, pull my underwear on.

By the time my car zooms along our country road, past cows and familiar barbed wire fences, I wonder how any woman cannot hold on to that suffering. How do we not allow it into our bodies? How do we release it from our wombs? If we do, are those women before us forgotten? I don't even know what those particulars are for my lineage, what their bodies have been through, other than guesses about the women I knew and know. It feels endless.

That night I transform into a tempest—my body cannot stop the sobs. Chris protests at first, thinks it another rage cycle, realizes it isn't, climbs the ladder, and places his body over mine. I don't curl into him. I don't actually need him in this moment. I lie on my back and stare at the ceiling as tears run down my cheeks, enough to wet the pillow. My wrecking ball heavy again. I hear myself call out to Pat-Pat and my father's mother, Grandmommy. My emotional connection to them never had time or space to develop.

But I call for them, for anyone else, for help.

I don't know if I can do this.

My pelvis weeps.

What if I can't heal myself—or feel really alive again? What if I pass that on to Eula? Now that I've opened to the possibility of healing, the possibility of not healing haunts me more. There are so many ailing women. There are so many. There have been many hopeful moments where I've thought, "This is it. I've resurfaced." And I don't know if I can hoist myself up again.

A wave of tenderness washes over me, for me, for all of us.

The body is made to heal.

The truth is I've never expected to fully heal, as if I'm destined for partial health forever.

I must expect to heal.

I wake to a bladder that has lost control again. My incontinence will reign for weeks, something released from scar tissue, a getting worse before getting better again. That afternoon, as I nestle Eula down for her nap and call forward women everywhere, lineage, ghosts, a message comes. In the other room, where no one is, I hear our woodstove creak open and then close with a firm sound.

~

Water is everywhere. Splash, splash in the bath, Eula splashes around in our utility sink. I've given her Mare's old ivory mirror. She scrubs it with a washcloth and explains to me that "Eula clean it." Then she pauses, gazes at herself in it. More scrub. Pause. Gaze. More scrub. Pause. Gaze. I stand, lean on the sink, and stretch out my calf muscles like a runner. We attract what we are. But we can remake what we are. We must have this option. *She* is pure source. She seems to have messages for me in every moment, or I just choose to make meaning from them.

At breakfast, she spilled her water glass onto the wood table on purpose.

"What are you doing, sweets?"

"Drawing," she said, as her finger moved through beads and smears of water.

"What are you drawing?" I asked.

"Woman. Long hair," she said, and I could see the long-haired woman she was making, could actually see her emerge from water spilled onto wood.

Now in her bath, she weaves water around the mirror her grandmother once gazed into as a girl. An hour later, she tires of the bath and hands me the mirror.

"Oooooo," she squeals, delighted by a warm towel and her mama's arms.

I pull the plug on the drain and we watch the water swirl down together.

"Goodbye, water, thank you, water," we say.

Thank you, water.

What would happen if I let my old water down back into the earth? My wounded-woman story gave me power when I felt powered down. Without it, I lose a few flashy items: the righteousness of being right and making my husband wrong, the permission and reason to vent, and a bunch of attention for being complicated and, therefore, interesting. Old story. Not helpful anymore.

My cells want to live into the next story.

They have gathered and staged the greatest protest of their lives.

Because beyond the story spreads a bursting green land.

The woman in labor lives there.

Oh, look at the space, look at the possibility.

My body need not be broken, right?

~

Eula turns two years old. Could it be? Green grass starts to poke up and snow stays in the faraway mountains. No great changes in my body. But my perception has changed. My period has come a week early. It's strange for me to be irregular, but the small dose of progesterone is re-regulating me.

After dinner, we walk up to her four-stone spot. It's her origin place. The grass is still matted down and a slight breeze greets us. She pulls her pants down, squats, and pees.

Then she balances on one of the rocks. Falls. Balances. Falls.

"Moon," she yells at the moon coming up. "Watch Eula do dis."

She commands the moon to watch.

She knows the moon.

She waves good night to it every evening.

As she continues to practice her balance, I sit in our meadow bowl surrounded by mountain ranges. We are small here. Somewhere elk bed down. Somewhere hawks coast over us. They don't think about the cycle because they have never removed themselves from the cycle. We have. We do it every day. There must be a way for modern women to live in a modern world and still hold on to the cycle. Our cycle might be the forgotten solution. I pull at grass and gather sticks around me to make something—wrap, fold, wrap, fold. What will it become? Eula scampers over to me, flops on my legs, watches me create, and when I'm done, I hold it up.

"There," I say.

"A woman," she responds.

"Yes," I say, and grab her to me. "It *is* a woman. How did you know?"

~

In my dream, Eula and I move upstream and uphill in a rowboat on a twisty road flooded to become a creek. The current grows thick and brown. The only way I can push us is by getting out of the boat to push it while doing breaststroke and relying on the power of my legs. Then another dream, in a public restroom, amniotic fluid pours out of me and keeps coming. I grab paper towels and try to mop it up but there is no end to it. I run outside to hide under a tree in a parking lot. Masses of people walk toward the building at dusk as violins fill the night air. "The orchestra," I hear people say. I must go back in to fess up but remain frozen, unsure of what to do.

In the real world, Eula starts to call out at night: "Where Mama go?"

In the real world, she bites her animals on the nose and then says, "Oh sorry," followed by a hug. I remember doing the same as a child—creating a pain so that you could soothe something.

In the real world, I see my body in the yoga-class mirror and love washes over me: *my* sweat, *my* red face, *my* strong butt, *my* dark hair, never before, the surge of such love. The viper within nods her head in approval. Could it be possible to let my body sadness be simply a moment in time that ended when I was thirty-six years old?

Let me get honest with myself.

In those early months of new motherhood, Chris held me from behind, licked tears from my eyes, reminded me it would pass, suggested that sleep deprivation affects mood more than we know. Any time I did my pelvic-floor exercises for a week straight, it helped, noticeably. My father wrote me a long letter sharing all the ways he *saw* me, a list of how he honored what I had been through, how proud he was of me for all of it because he had, over the years, grown from a man full of tension to one full of less tension who believes women are the answer to everything. My mother cooked for us and loved me through all my lash-outs. My doctor is also my friend. Chris woke with Eula as much as I did. He built us a house. I have freedom. I have freedom. I have freedom. She was born pink, not blue as the doctors expected. She was not compromised. My body has muscle memory. My body knows how to engage muscles. My body can remember how to heal. They tried to help me.

Be kind to others and myself.

Subterranean changes are the only way.

~

My brothers fly to Montana from other parts of the world. They are my limbs, I have always told people, and it's true. Something clicks back into place when we see each other. My parents offer to stay with Eula as she sleeps so we can sneak out to a cider house—me and the boys and my husband. I'm struck by what adults we are now. I sit across from them and watch the way they speak with such clarity. We are past youth. We have entered the meat of our lives.

Feminism comes up.

I don't remember exactly what gets said, something about how men often like when a woman acts soft or needs something. Peter loves being able to protect his wife, take care of her.

"That doesn't work for everyone," I say.

They all stare at me.

"Well, Chris," I continue, and notice acid in my throat, "you don't like it when I ask for help or need anything from you, if I appear weak."

"That's because you come at me with a spear when you make a request."

We choose to laugh. I choose not to latch on to my husband's comment, the way it shows his own unexpressed rage, his learned passiveness, his inability or lack of drive to help himself or seek counsel or be responsible to his own feelings. I tend to choose and then un-choose. My younger brother, Alex, feels kin to me, maybe because he's gay and feels marginalized too. Even he, though, says, "C'mon, Molly, it's the old dance between feminine and masculine." Across the gulf of a wooden table, I am the last woman standing. Even the men I trust live a hundred thousand miles away from me right now. They must be talking about goddess energy. It's the only way I can accept what I'm hearing.

As we walk out to the car, as dark descends over us, my fury slithers up, tells me that they know *nothing* about what it means to be a woman in need, and how complicated that is, or what it's like to have your body destroyed in the act of giving and sustaining human life. The whole thing is bullshit. For all their own woes, they don't ever do the personal work. They can never ever understand my situation in a felt-sense body way. Never.

I march onward and my arms start to shake.

Oh no. This is messy: trust your cycle, leave it till later, practice what you've learned, you can do it, take a breath.

We start to drive and I realize I am the woman driving the men who drank alcohol home. Hm. The urge within awakens. Maybe it's adrenaline or my older-sister tendency, but I cannot control it.

I hear my voice begin.

"Do any of you know what it's like to be broken and have no one help you? Do you know what it's like to be so zapped of energy you can't pick your baby up and then your husband walks out the door irritated at you? Do you know what it feels like to not know if you can ever run again without urine pouring out of you? Have you ever experienced anything close to this? And do you know it's not only me? It's many women, women all over the fucking world. Do you have *any* idea?"

"Whoa, Molly," Alex says from the backseat. "This is intense. It sounds like you are in a lot of pain, but this is a lot."

"Yeah, it's a lot," I scream. "Welcome to my life."

Chris audibly breathes next to me in the dark, protects himself by staring out the window.

"Are you blaming Chris?" Peter asks. "It sounds like you are talking about him and he's in this car right now. This is really inappropriate. You need to stop."

Oxygen flees our car.

Don't you dare tell me to stop.

My mouth, though, stops.

I remember words, phrases, hurtful controlling ones from my younger brothers right around my puberty, when I became a woman, and later: *Yeah everyone in this family is beautiful, except for Molly. You're really letting yourself go. You used to be like a model, what happened?* I've never dwelled on them, but now they snap onstage. No reverence for a girl becoming a woman. Old teases between siblings. Ha ha.

They get out at the cabin.

We inch the car back to our house.

"Sorry, babe," I beg of Chris, who says nothing back to me. With bed covers over my head, the sludge becomes a hard stone in my belly. I am certain I have destroyed my marriage and my sisterhood. My only option is to hide.

No sleep.

No chance of sleep. I get up before dawn and leave. My pee pours out of me. The link between my rage/sadness and my incontinence is unmistakable. My car chugs up into the mountains, past so many trees. Suddenly, a female elk emerges from the woods, tall and stately at the edge of the road. She wakes me. We lock eyes as I continue, up, up, up with no plan other than not to return for hours.

At the top of nowhere, I slouch down into my car seat and let my sorrows out.

I don't have energy to walk into the forest.

Hours later, when cars start to approach with people eager for a weekend hike, I buckle my seatbelt in the early pale sun and descend back to the valley floor. Me, a sepia image no one in this current world can recognize. Not ready to see anyone, I park my car on our dirt road and sneak up and around to the top of our hill.

My body crumbles down on the four-stone spot.

Facedown, arms out, and I release it all down into this Mother Earth, all of it, every last drop of me, scent of loam, turn my sludge to loam. Round the hurt out. I can feel Eula's words below, *Where Mama go?* Oh god. A tiny ant with wings catches my attention, the way it walks up and down blades of grass, pauses, not sure where to go, but slow and fast and purposeful. My brothers have offered me a shovel. My gender work is not done. Later this afternoon, Chris and I will call Janice from our gray hatchback. When she asks how we are doing, a scream will erupt from my mouth. It's my scream for all ages, a scream with no shame because there is so much shame.

But now, small black birds have landed nearby, so close, so long I've been here I become one of the flock and when at last my head rises, the whole earth shudders as they fly away and up.

~

What I learn: We cannot separate a culture's treatment of women from that same culture's treatment of the earth. The theory and study behind the connection is academic, ecological, and displayed in our everyday moments in homes across the world. When I scream into the earth, she hears me and has the remarkable tender strength to hold whatever comes out of me. Somewhere, in England, France, all over Africa, all over Asia, all over everywhere, ancient stone goddesses hold vulvas open in celebration, an offering of the divine, a passageway.

The earth also offers itself as a passage for anyone.

Come into my arms, it says.

You can rest here.

~

The early summer nights wake me up—all owls, coyotes, wind, some sound like crickets but less dense. My brothers have left. Chris and I have made our way back to each other. One evening, in bed, our sex heat builds, and light starts to spread out and up from the base of my tail, as it always does, and then a flash. Men. Many men. Smothering. Me smothered.

"Please stop," I say, "*now.*" He does. Arousal dissolves. Release halts. With a *whomp*, my root becomes a vacuum, no movement, no sound, no sense of me. I don't know yet that it will stay this way for almost two months.

We lie in the darkness.

He puts a hand on my shoulder.

"I don't know what just happened," I say. "Strange, flash, strange past-life flash of me, but not me. Strange. It's not you. It's other men. I don't know."

"It's okay," he assures me.

"Maybe I can get back into it," I say, feeling bad even though I know I shouldn't feel bad and he doesn't expect me to get back into anything. We drift into sleep and my dream takes us on a descending elevator. The belt securing Chris snaps and he falls to the deepest hardest floor, lands on his head. I fly down and pull him into my arms. This still-alive but severely broken man becomes a boy, and I am yelling at people to get the quickest plane to Bangkok, and then the boy becomes my brother Alex and then my brother Peter and then other boys I don't know, so many boys in my woman arms. These men. They are not so harmful. They are harmed too.

In the morning, I stand barefoot in the bathroom alone.

The sun lights up trees outside.

I touch between my legs—strange vacant black hole of space.

All my gender rage makes and unmakes itself in my pelvis.

Of course. I have been a woman who believed men would hurt her body for the simple reason she was female. This belief is not my own—it comes from a collective truth, came to me in a flood from ancestors I cannot name, perhaps comes to every woman that way. The man in the elevator did hurt me. But he was one man. The men in my family are not *that* man. I often tell friends if only women populated the world, I would spread out my arms, sway my hips, footfall my way into dance, and inhabit my sensuality, sexuality, and womanhood with no fear.

None.

I do understand the complex biology of it. I do understand the beauty of the male-female dance, but I cannot ignore the deep history of violation toward women. We are capable of evolving into a new connection. Just because men might be programmed to spread their seed doesn't mean men should violate and disrespect. Just because women might be programmed to grow babies doesn't mean every woman must grow a baby.

The one person who can create that well of safety is me.

It is a shedding process. As we make breakfast, Chris sees the analyzing in my eyes. He knows I tend toward leaden truths. He pulls my face close to his and smiles.

"Babe, I know you had a past-life flash last night," he says, and squints love at me, "but it might not help you to relive it all day long."

I laugh.

"Yes, true," I say.

My practical man is good for me.

~

On the first of June, Eula finds a dead vole near our garden bed.

"Oh-p," she says, and squats down to investigate.

"Bru must have gotten it," I explain.

"It's be okay, though," she says with a nod. I nod back. Yes, even though it's dead, the vole is still okay. Bare hands. We push dirt up over the vole. We bury it and allow the moist dirt under our fingernails. It is her first burial.

We all must bury an old way so a new way may grow up.

I am learning this about my life.

She will learn this about her own.

I watch my daughter, industrious under the gray sky. I will no longer make choices that compromise my own energy. I will take an uncharacteristic deep pause for the summer. Can the summer be a healing one? Eula will toddle back to the vole every day for over a week, on her own, to check in, a vigil for the dead creature.

The days tumble forward.

I'm off progesterone with Holcomb's approval. It has done what it needs to do. I toss the packet of unused troches in the trash.

My body starts to ovulate with the full moon.

My cycle matched to a natural cycle—again, at last.

As we make rice pasta and salads and bison, as we meet friends at the park and I roll down a hill and don't break, as baby robins hurl themselves out of nests into the world, my ovary releases an egg.

Eggs appear in one of my dreams. In an underground bar, a faceless bearded man, the oldest and kindest of grandfathers, approaches me. What does he want? I'm leery. He opens a paper towel to reveal a tiny, bloody egg. It's from my ovary. Why does a man have my egg? He reads my mind.

"I have your egg because I want to show you what they look like," he says to me.

Then he hands me another paper towel. It is heavy with all of my eggs. They look like rosehips. They are all here. They were in me in my mother in her mother in her mother until the beginning of time. Holcomb appears, glances over my shoulders, and gasps at the beauty. She didn't know they looked like that.

My seeds. My possibilities.

Multitudes.

Who Chose a Cause and a Person

As my youth evaporated, I sensed what many other women sense
then. There was something my body wanted to do, if I chose it. Not
yet. No baby yet. We had been together for almost ten years. At
some point, marriage or a form of deeper commitment would happen. I didn't need to rush anything. But the tunnel had presented
itself—another passageway. You will have choices to make soon.
You must narrow your options and come to know that a boundary
is not a roadblock but an open door. You will become a more adult
woman.

My parents, open to all, did not suggest how *it* should be. They
knew I would choose what I wanted. They had handed me that supreme freedom at birth. Chris and I moved together to New York
City. New adventure. Why not? Surrounded by concrete. My first
desk job ever. No window. Corridors of hallways and skyscrapers and
so little sky. Gin and tonics after work. Working with words and
authors. Mind alive. Body stagnant. Sit at a computer all day long.

Within two weeks, shooting pains down my legs.

Within five weeks, deep ache in my chest.

But the body adjusts. My senses sharpened as much as they dulled.

Be alert. Tune out.

I liked the city.

I liked that it gave me, gave everyone, an audience, even if that audience never paid attention. On a packed subway, with the usual smell of trash everywhere, we made our way one evening to a Halloween party. Chris had dressed as a shepherd with a wooden stick and very short shorts. For six months, I had watched herds of women, all types of women. My childhood frustration about the world and femaleness amplified in this setting. I had costumed myself into the Depo-Provera birth control shot—shiny aluminum foil hat with a coat hanger coming straight out the top, and on my back hung a list of all the horrific side effects and a mention that a man had invented this, along with all other forms of hormonal birth control that, yes, gave a woman critical social freedom but could also imprison her body. That's what I had read about and witnessed in almost all of my friends, and in myself. But few people knew or admitted to it. It was tricky because it went against what most of my New York people believed. To say hormonal birth control was problematic could sound like you weren't a feminist—which wasn't the case for me. It came from a deep feminism within me. It was a long spiel. It mattered to me. The nuance. The birth control pill gave women ownership of their bodies at a critical time in history. I wanted to think about a new kind of ownership. It was time for a better option that connected women to instead of divorcing them from their bodies. Why did no one talk about this shit? Men or women?

I got some stares.

I got a lot of stares before the eve was over.

By that point, charting my menses had become a daily part of my life. I could tell anyone what my cervical fluid typically looked like on day seven, fourteen, and eighteen of my cycle. Most mainstream doctors gave me the rude *Wow, aren't you involved with your body* glare of shock. I poured my menstrual blood into the soil of our eighteen apartment plants.

Life veered on messy because a bomb had fractured within me. Gender rage. Every moment of my life had suddenly clicked into position and I understood the inequality and violence had been acute, for eons, for every woman—and I wasn't even remotely close to the worst-off one. It hurt every moment. It wouldn't go away. I had some awareness that it might take years to extract every last piece of shrapnel. When men whistled at me on the street, I shot them death stares. Why did they feel they could control me? I became reactive. My anger toward men was my anger toward history and toward the masculine predator in me. My anger toward women who weren't angry about it was my anger toward the feminine in me. I defended myself before ever having to actually defend myself. Once, and only once, I tried something different, something I had witnessed Lauren and a few other women doing. When the construction workers grinned at me and whistled, I swept my head back toward them and answered, "Thank you," with a big wide smile on my face, swung my hips, and continued down the street, inhabited by a woman who had never emerged before. It would have been so easy to greet them that way again and again. But that move had taken all my focus. I wasn't ready to let anyone off the hook.

Once there was an angry woman; one day she would transform.

Into what, though?

I wanted to rediscover my athletic self. Under gray buildings, among the press of other humans, I tested her—tried to kickbox, then found my way outdoors, swam races in a murky river full of used condoms, cycled out of the city and almost one hundred miles in one stretch every week, ran my flat feet in long circles around busy parks.

I said it was to be strong.

It was.

It was also my secret hope to morph for good into a thin woman. I burned a truckload of calories, but none of the fat around my hips went away. I couldn't yet connect that what we feel presents in the body. Anger, it is said, adheres to the body as unnecessary flesh, as disease, as bloat, as inflamed cells.

My parents lived nearby and came to watch my races. Their young adult selves flowered up around us often, my father with his mustache, my mother in her colorful scarves. During our few years there, I wanted to ingest my own mother, absorb her into me, but couldn't out of my own limitation. We once saw a theatre play together. Tucked into the plush chair, she appeared serene, easy, as usual, despite her recent shoulder surgery. The story broke something open in me, as art does, but I willed the tears away. Afterward, spit back onto the slick streets, we walked through dark sky, glitter, and light flashes every-where, and in the distance, drilling.

"Those men, drilling," she said.

"Could be women," I said. She, my elegant mother, had my arm because she always has my back. I should have had her arm. She, the elder, was the broken one, and yet, she had rarely needed attention for her brokenness. We exchanged casual banter, me so monotone, clogged up with emotion. I would walk her to the train station before catching a cab, a once-a-month luxury, uptown to my apartment. And because I didn't know what else to do, I complained about how late I would be to get home, how much work awaited me on my desk to-morrow. We began flailing our arms for a cab. No luck. Where were the fucking cabs? She let go of my arm and lurched her whole body, with shoulder brace, into the street.

"Mom!" I yelled.

She knew she could get run over. She would stop at nothing to hail her daughter a cab, her arm extended out, her determination enough to solidify my self-disgust in this moment. Before I could step forward, replace her, usher her back to the sidewalk, she yanked open a yellow door, and fast, because that's what the city requires of a person, I slid into the vehicle, and our eyes met briefly until I was off, jetting up toward my home. She would walk two more blocks to her train. Alone. This would not bother her.

The smell of plastic and stale air made my anonymity known. I allowed the years of gratitude and shame to burst from me—another lost chance to love my mother how she deserved to be loved. Heavy heaving, sobs, choking, another lost chance, another lost chance, an-other lost chance, so many lost chances. Nothing a cabbie hadn't seen before.

It was a real-deal lost chance.

Soon after, Chris and I quit our jobs and moved out West.

We landed on land owned by my parents with no foreshadow it would become our home. The return to nature requests a return to body. You cannot avoid it. Hawk, bear, mountain lion, fox, elk, eagle, deer, marmot, creek, mountain, trees, canyons, valleys, clouds.

I could breathe.

I hadn't expected to meet a breed of people who had chosen mountains above all else. Every activity relied on, was sustained by, depended upon an intensity reflected in the high peaks surrounding us. No one went on *walks*. Friends invited each other on last-minute twenty-mile runs, backcountry ski adventures through avalanche territory, mountain bike journeys of uphill switchbacks for the first long leg. I couldn't accept any of these invitations, even when someone like Holcomb assured me she didn't care how fast we went or how far we got. Nothing had changed in my physical body. But upon entrance, I felt again like the fat friend who couldn't keep up with anyone.

My belief was such a limitation.

I had wanted to be called into my body like this since girlhood.

But I glanced once and chose no. I heard myself making a case for a culture of movement that wasn't so "driven" or masculine, but really that was my way of protecting myself from the hurt of it. At a clothing swap, as women who had become dear to me danced around a pile of size 2, 4, 6, 8 discards, one well-meaning friend approached me, saying, "These, Molly, *these*," with a pair of pants she thought were big enough to fit me. I smiled at her and left my body, floated up to the ceiling to gaze out the high windows until it was over and I could leave.

Hiker. That's what I became, and that's it.

I could have gone for it—started up, pushed myself, learned, stepped into the adventurous me. There were so many Patagonia-model outdoor women here. I just could not fit. It was less humiliating to cut myself from the team but, in the end, the pain of being separate from it would be constant.

Even deeper when it felt, later, like the last chance I never took.

I began to see my body as broken somehow.

But my body was not and did not want to be broken. The body never does.

Meanwhile, I read books about the pelvic bowl even though the pelvic bowl was no issue for me. What was that sacred place? How could I know it better? When a friend had prolapse trouble after the birth of her daughter, she told me about the sex toy that doubled as a tool to help her heal. I bought it too to strengthen my already-strong pelvic tone. When Chris asked about it for sex, I said, "Maybe, but probably not; it's meant for deep personal woman work."

I had to be that serious. My pelvis was sending me a message. Listen. Listen to me. Listen because all the answers, all the grief, the explosive joy, the need to protect, the creation, the want, it all lives here, between your hips.

After our wedding, we took a few years to organize a honeymoon. I picked my clothes carefully—red blouse, short black dress, white striped pants. This was my chance to feel good, an actual pulled-together woman. My mother had glowed on her honeymoon. She wore scarves and dresses around an island jungle. She propped her foot on the steps of a bungalow and gave her steady gaze to a camera.

We traveled around the south of Spain, where ancient people had once coexisted: Muslims, Jews, and Christians under olive trees sharing ideas with one another. We absorbed what the morning light might have done back then. It might have spread across the river, circled around a building, scraped away the darkness, until it reached a red tiled floor and leapt up to shine over the tops of heads leaned together in discourse. Over *patatas bravas* and wine, I watched my husband.

When you choose a person, you choose whom you will dream *and* struggle with.

That is the choice.

In a small mountain town, we checked into our tiny hotel, ate asparagus, and ended up back in our pale green room for a nap. The gauze of no responsibility settled over us, until I woke, one eye, then the other, and there, my bare legs, an angle, such ugly legs, these legs of mine, not what should have been on my honeymoon. Not what should have been. Not what should be. I wasn't the beautiful bride I wanted to be. I didn't even know I had wanted to be a beautiful bride. I had fought against the image my entire life.

With the knowing, a wave approached. It swamped me, un-lodged a pit somewhere in the nethermost part of me, and tossed it around, bruising me all over again. Choking sounds, a weeping beyond me, convulsions. I crawled away from my still-asleep husband to the bathroom. I welcomed the pelting of a shower. The waves grew and then subsided and washed the pit out, some sense that an old force had passed out of me, not for good, but the start of it.

Me curled up in the bathtub. Wet. Glistening like a newborn.

I wore shorts and walked the countryside for the next two days. No more apologies, I thought.

Ground

My long pause over the summer means simple focus: move, eat, nature, love each other. I want to arrive on the continent—no more unwanted pee—without having to trek across a dangerous and slippery glacier. Is there a way to effort less, to be gentle? Warmth calms me. Summer is my season.

"Mama, sing 'She'll Be,'" Eula asks.

My mom has taught her the song "She'll Be Coming 'Round the Mountain." She remembers songs I forgot existed. At least four times a day, outside on the ragged green grass, inside on our floor couch, Eula asks me to cross my legs so she can sit on my foot and bounce her way into the song.

What will she be; what will we be; what will I be? The other day, I inched my car up the driveway after a long solo hike in the mountains. It's my intention for the summer: to process less and embody more, to play, to act *as if* my body is already healthy, as if I am beautiful and can wear shorts and not be shy about my more-plump legs, as if I can be kind. Eula ran fast across the grass/dirt to me, leapt into my arms, hugged me, and then pulled my face to hers, so close, and took me in, almost made a move to ingest the whole of me.

~

At my new pelvic therapist's office, I sit on a brown massage table and tell her about my incontinence. It's better but not over, linked very much to my cycles, worse before menstruating. Also, there's the small prolapse and I might like to have another baby one day.

"Okay," she says, "tell me what you want to be able to do again, what movement, what—"

"I want," I interrupt, "to leap, dance, climb trees, run down the driveway with my daughter. I don't need to run a marathon, but I want to be able to go on a fifteen-mile hike and feel good at the end, not like my organs are protruding out of my vagina, not sticky with urine."

She beams at me, nods with the vigor of a boxer before a match. I'm amused that her mouth is so full of joy about all of this. At least I am far more accepting of her than I would have been a year or two ago. It's possible. Not a problem. Not a problem at all. We can fix that for you. No, surgery is definitely not necessary. Really? Yep, we'll get you feeling great and back together.

Those words don't compute. She is so sure.

It is a foreign language I don't know yet.

Somewhere, later, on a forest walk, Holcomb and I stare at each other and make a collective decision. Let's not connect over our brokenness anymore. It's so easy to do so. This is what women do. But it tires us now. It is *enough*, we say. I don't know what her body tells her in this moment. Mine screams, "Revolution!!!!" We make sure to assure each other of exceptions. Of course, there will be times. She is my doctor. We are friends. We became mothers together. Nothing is absolute.

But woundology is sneaky.

Strapped to our backs, our daughters absorb the sun, perhaps also our words.

Do they hear us?

This is where time speeds up, because when healing accelerates, time hitches a ride and then spins out of the molasses and into a space so vast and thin there is no resistance. Nothing to push against.

~

What I learn: My purple kidneys attach to my bladder—and that bladder looks much like a leather purse. Imagine the beauty and design of it. Pelvic *dysfunction* is often attributed to already-weak pelvic muscles, but how we define *weak* is a common misunderstanding. We think of weak as not strong. Many women have a "strong" pelvic floor, often too tight, rigid. It may be a form of protection and this, in effect, can cause weakness. The ideal for pelvic health, like life, is to find a place of supple and strong flexibility. Many body-workers believe a misaligned pelvis can be directly linked to postpartum depression or rage.

Makes sense to me after everything.

What we don't speak is a curse. Our collective history wants a full-powered speaker system. To speak it is a hurdle, but *how* to speak it is the greater challenge. We don't want to misdirect it to wound others, yes; but more importantly, how can we speak it so the healing within us can actually take place? This continues to be my biggest learning. It's my practice now. Spewing feels good in the moment but it does not do the work of sustainable deep release. That work, for women or men, comes from an attunement to the feminine.

In our weedy pond, Eula recoils in my arms, unsure of the slimy grasses for her first open-water swim. Goose bumps creep along our naked torsos. She grips my nipple. The sky spreads a pale blue. I tell her the pond is magic.

"It is?"

"It is."

Minutes later, she splashes and paddles the grasses toward her, invites them to rest like snakes on her body. We are covered in grass snakes. I scrunch my toes in the loam beneath and send my energy down just as I draw it up into me. This has to be a daily remembrance. The earth can instruct me in the feminine. Eula has begun to communicate, at length, about what she remembers—when we crawled through our fence last autumn as cottonwood leaves fell, how she cried out, "Need Mama, need big hug," in the night and how

Mama came, when Holcomb checked Mama's vulva under the big white sheet and Mama was okay.

I don't know how she remembers events from six months or even a year ago.

"*You* remember," I coo at her.

She leans forward, as she does, to touch her forehead to mine in recognition.

"Mama loves you," she says, as the grasses sway around us.

By *you*, she means me and her.

~

Every summer Wednesday, I trade half of my workday for a long solo hike. I read for my clients at night. The mountains embrace me into whatever pulses: rain, heat, silence. For over two years, almost three, I have not exercised fully. I haven't been able to move without discomfort or grief about the discomfort. It's been easier to avoid movement. I'm done with avoidance. My legs move over rocks, up steep, across creeks, and I change my thoughts from *My body is broken* to *My body heals itself with ease.*

Practice required.

My question evolves.

When will my body heal?

To not effort is still a stretch for me. I believe I must lift weights. I must eat arugula and chicken and avoid sugar, gluten, and eating chocolate in the privacy and peace of my car. I must sweat. I must transmute my anger when I am triggered by something Chris does or does not do. I must conserve my emotional energy. I must keep my writing workshops afloat and reinvent a few. I must do yoga, not sit and stare at the wall during Eula's one-hour nap. I must use my evenings for my own writing and then rouse myself at five forty-five every morn to meditate and, at least three days a week, drink a green smoothie before driving to the hot springs at dawn.

It's hard to do it all, but I must, must, must—in order to be healed.

On these woods walks, I construct bubbles of possibility and plan my schedule, bubble up, bubble up. I can do it. My friends start to hear me talk about resilience. We saw our overly resilient mother and grandmothers package and bury the hard emotions, then decided we would be wise and feel and process every small emotion that surfaced in whatever way we wanted. Let's be sad and broken and angry together because that is real. Let's be real. Let's be deep and unmasked. I'm not the only one of my female friends with intense rage: other women with fists slammed against glass windows, phones thrown, screams hurled, punches into walls, whole-body shudders and wails. We've revealed these moments to each other, afraid at first and then relieved to know we are not alone. It is not our solitary experience. I hear us discussing how hard the ubiquitous *it* always is. Pendulum swing. Necessary.

But we didn't know how to reframe it: how to feel the feelings *with* a resilience and practice of connecting to cycles. There's an art there. It's old too. Women long ago knew how to engage ritual and move energy.

That knowing is in all of us.

I want to invite her back into me.

Look at her muscled legs. Look at the way her tree-bark hair falls thick, loose around her shoulders. Between her hips, a red glow no one can take from her. Nothing in her way. At the top of my climb, I consider her and sit in a peephole cave made of rock. The hike has a different name but I've renamed it Womb Rock. From here, layers of unbroken green mountains.

Some days Eula calls her vulva "my body." I don't correct her language.

Some days I wear a pad; some days I don't.

Some days I pee on myself, especially on the downhill; some days I don't.

I also go to a place I've named Deep Lake, a cold blue large mountain lake. I sneak around to a pine-needled stone beach and strip my sweaty clothes off, plunge in, down, into what feels like a pelvic bowl, wise, watery, calm. My limbs go numb. I kick around, float, swim back to shore and lie naked on a rock.

"I don't want to be a woman disconnected from her pelvis," I explain to Chris.

"I am falling in love with the female form," I say.

"Good, babe," he says.

As cottonwoods and firs fan down over me—they so unaffected—every new thought feels like a spark from an old thought. Over weeks, the earth shoots a deeper awareness up through my feet. It settles between my legs. I can hear it. But I won't be able to receive it into my body until cool weather moves in and leaves start to blow, fall, and tumble from trees.

~

Over cantaloupe and eggs, I stare into Eula's eyes with a serious love. Bright sun blinds our wood kitchen table. I communicate without words that I love her this much. She smiles and spreads her arms wide to show me that *Mama loves her this much.* We are humans becoming animals who need no words to express.

~

Three families. Five kids under age seven. Two or three miles. Camping gear. Bear country. Fathers haul double packs or pull a packed hiking stroller from behind. Toddlers scramble over rocks, dawdle, run and then get swooped up and carried by mothers who also wear packs on backs, one of whom, Holcomb, is also pregnant with her second daughter. We have somehow become this intense. I don't tell anyone how proud I am for not peeing while carrying Eula on my belly and a pack on my back, fifty pounds total. Eula says it for me. "Good job, Eula," she speaks to herself with each pull over a tree root, each run down the trail toward her friends, each run back to me. Mosquitoes and food and dogs and a campfire and the distraction of getting kids asleep in tents so we may catch some adult time which doesn't happen because everyone is mostly exhausted and there is so much to say and so little breath to say it with.

Twenty-four hours later, on our hike out, I hold my bladder up with each footfall.

I don't care if anyone sees.

I must tend.

I hear myself notice that I'm the largest woman on this adventure, and then I hear myself say, *Old story, keep walking.* My prolapse is much worse after the hike yesterday, but despair doesn't lure me over to her cozy bed. I become practical. Over two years ago, when we first understood my pelvic floor was an issue, Chris suggested I treat it like a broken ankle. Do your exercises, and it will get better. He became an alien to me then. We were talking about my root, my woman essence, not an ankle. But now I've gone through a passage of my own creation and will do my pelvic-floor exercises and all will be well. It's okay. It's okay. It's okay.

We emerge from the woods feral and missing one dog.

Fathers go back to look for the dog. Mothers wrangle children into shade, break out leftover food, bags of granola, seaweed, what else do we have. We have them, these little whole people who delight in their scratches, tangled hair, bruised knees, faces smudged with dirt, earth.

I am done with my own catastrophe.

Please may I be.

~

The whole world changes in July—trees reach out, grass blades sturdy, creeks full of birds. Cottonwoods have shed white cotton all over lawn. On the cabin's porch, my mom and I sit and watch naked Eula. She waters the potted geraniums.

"Pick off the dead flowers like this, Eula," my mom shows her.

We prune. We are such worker women when we want to be.

When we step off the porch back toward our house, summer caresses us more.

Overhead, one, two hawks fly. The creek bumbles along, a sound we don't know we are hearing because it is constant. Heat, my beloved heat, imprints ease on me, on us. Barefoot. Bees buzz everywhere. Eula knows to let the bees be. She struts through the warm grass, then starts to sing, "Bye, Mare, I love you, Mare, bye, Mare!" Her nude strut turns to dance turns to jog as we meet the gravel driveway and continue on. My mother waves from her kitchen door and off we go.

This scene. Can I preserve it? It has all felt so hard, but this is easy—this grandmother, mother, daughter scene on a hot midsummer day. I wonder if I was born a person who wills everything to be hard.

There are many partial truths. The world is made of these partial truths.

My daily ministration is to ask my feminine side, the left, to lead my masculine side, the right. Does it mean something that all of my challenges, small and large, are on the right side of my body—right ankle, right hip, right pelvic bowl, right eye. It has worked to be powerful. It is tired. We were never meant to be symmetrical, though.

I re-pattern.

My left hand holds my right hand.

My left leg leads up the ladder instead of my usual right leg.

My left pelvis, please teach right pelvis how to hold herself, how to open but not collapse. It is another new conversation with my body—not an intention written down in a journal, but an actual physical holding and change.

Eula flits around the house these days clutching her bear Mo-Mo and whispering, "I've got you, Mo-Mo, I'm here," into his ear, a phrase she repeats and repeats because she's heard it from me. Her repetition offers it back to me.

"I've got you," my left side says to my right side.

And then on the Fourth of July, while my man and daughter sleep, I lead my parents up the hill at dark to watch fireworks. It takes your full animal self to walk at night in Montana. Our eyes sift shadows from movement from wind. We sit on grass and gaze out over a valley gone primordial. Sounds echo far away. It looks like war. It could also be heaven. I hold my arms and think about how hair, skin, nails, consciousness are made up of where you live. The cells of the earth beneath my butt and the air around me make up the cells of me. Bru leans his long tiger body closer to me. In this company, I become a girl who watches. I am on the search for models. There are teachers everywhere. My parents talk and, at the exact instant my neck turns, an eagle coasts low right behind us in the dark. No one else sees her. No one else hears.

~

We've made a long effort at a very gradual teaching of how to sleep—rocking to holding to patting on back to sitting next to bed to sitting near doorway. It has worked, but then we hit these impasses where Eula is getting a tooth or growing and our tidy plan unravels and we're back to one of us sleeping on a worn-out mattress in the hallway next to her room. When she wakes up, we tell her we can't go outside until the sun rises. She watches for the sun out the window and then yells, "Yay! Sun is up! Yay!" She's been clingy lately, unlike herself, wanting to be sure that I will come back when I go away. So now I just lie down in her twin bed—for naps and night—and let her tweak my nipple, my arm heavy over her body, our faces pressed sweaty together as she whispers, "Mama is here," and I repeat, "I'm here," and we fall asleep together and eventually, twenty minutes later, I wake and sneak out.

I mostly love it.

Instead of reading sleep books, I am doing what my body likes.

"Do whatever is easiest for you," Chris says. I don't have to do anything but be all snuggles with my daughter. When I feel myself loving it too much, I counsel myself that she won't be a fifteen-year-old who needs to hold on to her mother's nipple. This will end. This, right now, allows me to keep some energy. But I also pay attention to an intuition that, sooner or later, I'll have to wean her from this ease too—and maybe that will be even more exhausting.

At this point, though, I give in.

"Why?" everyone asks.

Because I want to reorganize my relationship to effort.

~

One Wednesday, I go up to Deep Lake with a friend. Normally, I would wear my black nylon skirt with no underwear. It's how I play these days and how women once sat, with vulva to earth. But I'm not alone. In the presence of someone else, I wear pants.

As our feet pound the ground, we talk.

"I don't think I'm all that connected to my body," I say.

"I don't think that's true about you," she says.

"It isn't true. I don't know why I said it."

We walk on, over rocks, roots.

"What I mean is," I continue, "I don't feel I have a right to say I'm connected to my body because I feel fat. I think I have a core belief that fat people aren't connected to their bodies. I know this is wrong, incorrect, mean."

A rocket has launched out of me.

I don't remember what she says.

She listens, though.

I listen too, to the oldest parts of me as they surface and leave and travel beyond in me and eventually lose steam. Once that rocket makes it past our galaxy, away, I start to make specific changes at home. I cut underwire out of my three bras. I ask a dentist to remove the metal lingual bar from behind my bottom teeth. I am done with metal on my body. I schedule a haircut and a bikini wax. I don't care about the cost anymore. After a shower, I brush my hair and Eula mimics me with her brush—our heads cocked to the side, slow strokes. Then she shows me how Mare does it in fast motions, a fluff from behind. So this is how we learn movement. When I start to pull my hair up into a loose bun, the only way I ever wear it, Eula stares at me.

"Don't put pony in, Mama," she says.

Okay, I will let my hair down.

At bedtime now, Eula crawls around my bare legs to get comfortable in bed. I sit surrounded by her animals and tell her it's okay, no more nipple, but she can be close to my legs. She clutches them, as if they will protect her.

She came from these legs.

Her benediction for them becomes my own.

Okay, I will let my legs out.

I have so often heard older women say something like, "Oh that's back when I was skinny, when I was beautiful . . ." They engage in a grief of change. I know that grief. I can make comments about back when I could run and cartwheel. But my beauty story is a grief of never having the experience. It's one thing to have it and lose it. It's another grief if you never had it. And it's a deeper clenching grief when you understand that you actually did have it but you never let yourself feel it.

Okay, I will celebrate this body I have.

~

Eula continues to ask me to sing "She'll Be." The more often the words come out of my mouth, the more I remember how when we think we've become something "new," life gives us a hurdle, small or oversized, to deepen our unfolding. Maybe my fear has woken up again. Maybe it has wet feathers and wants to dry them off. But time and a series of choices still seem to have catapulted me toward health. I'm midair. I can see where I'm headed.

Toward the end of August, nausea returns to me.

I don't know where it is coming from.

I'm not pregnant again.

"So, do you think it's strange that I'm feeling nauseous just like I did when I was first pregnant with Eula?" I ask Chris. "I mean that was almost *exactly* three years ago."

"Huh," he says, as he makes his coffee, "what else could it be?"

"The symptoms are identical. I can't tolerate the smell of coffee grounds or burnt bread. I don't want to eat much."

"I don't know then."

"Or," I say, "it might be the new adrenal herbs." With another recent test, Holcomb has told me my adrenals are very low. She wouldn't say flatlined, but almost. In some cases with these levels, she would consider cortisol. Adrenals are linked to thyroid. She explained the adrenals are the car tires and the thyroid is the engine. If the car tires are flat, pressing on the gas gets you nowhere. Point is, even though low adrenals is common for new parents, it shouldn't go untended to. She asked whether I've had enough energy to get through my day. I didn't know what to say. I make do. Other than herbs, adrenals heal with routine and ease and low stress and not a whole lot of effort— like a vacation.

Exercise needs to be tapered too.

Nothing strenuous.

It occurs to me to be frustrated. I'm suddenly capable of exercise because my incontinence is better but now can't exercise because of adrenals. I walk up our hill and stomp my feet around for half an hour, punch the ether like someone who knows what she's doing. That helps. No need for melodrama.

Eula sits on the counter and licks paprika from the spice bottle.

"Want some, Mama?" she asks.

"Sure, sweets, sure."

~

What I learn: The adrenals sit above each kidney in the middle of the lower back. One is triangular and the other looks like a half-moon—both are the size of an infant's palm. They make many hormones, like cortisol, a name semi-common for most laypeople. Cortisol fluctuates in response to stress and can affect immune function, blood sugar handling, and inflammation, thereby affecting metabolism.

Many of us have taxed adrenals.

Our lives don't accommodate slowness and space.

I'm on that mission now.

~

Holcomb and I take our girls to the hot springs. We wiggle them into swimsuits and slip together into the shallow pool to find warm water and steps for them to play and test themselves on. They love to jump in our arms. The big leap. My pelvis tells me it is heavy and ready to bleed. I know it'll come tomorrow. The cycle of it feels good to me. Holcomb is almost seven months pregnant with another girl.

"How do you feel?" I ask.

"You know," she laughs, and she means not *you* as me, but *you* as all of us.

We talk. The girls splash, so close to being able to swim solo but not yet. We wonder aloud how her still-nursing daughter will do when a newborn wants the boob. Who knows? I tell her how I've been going to Eula in the middle of the night when she calls out, "Where's Mama?" I can't not go; I end up sleeping in her bed. I get it, she says. The breast is still a focus for us, though milk stopped what feels like ages ago. I tell Holcomb about this morning when I woke to a gray light and Eula was already sitting up. She ran her fingers slowly from breast to breast, down my sternum to my belly button and back up, like a blessing or honoring. I opened my eyes and we smiled at each other. I asked her whether she remembered how she came out of me. "Out your vulva, Mama," she said.

"They know so much," Holcomb says, and we laugh.

"Can you believe you're going to do that again?"

"It feels so far away."

So much feels far away and yet it's not.

I too am getting closer to my laboring woman.

I can feel her speaking to me, even though I've stopped going to the pelvic therapist. Our insurance didn't cover it and the bills became mountains. But it gave me hope that my pelvic bowl can restore itself.

Two hours pass and, surrounded by steam, we become red-faced, all of us. As we lumber up and out of the water, we enter the world again—wet, slick, warm, the blood of us pump, pump, pumps.

~

My mom and I pull apart a roast chicken. She yanks it apart. In the bright light of my kitchen, I stand beside her and cringe. I've never been adept with dead animal parts.

"It's easy," she says as we toss carrots, celery, onion and all the chicken parts into a pot of water. I've made broth before but not with any sort of knowledge or repetition. She is teaching me. People pay her to show them how to make a pork lemongrass meatball, green soup, or pear cheesecake, and then how to invent their own creation. I'm letting go of my limitations—too domestic, too my mother, too quaint, too oppressed women throughout history.

Now my interest grows like wildfire.

I will un-oppress myself by feeding my body well.

As we skim gray stuff from the boiling water, I am sure a shift is happening: onset of fall, cottonwood leaves turn yellow, amber, Molly makes a broth, emboldened. Four days later, I make another roast chicken, chicken broth, ghee, sweet tahini balls, pumpkin soufflé, chia seed pudding, and arugula pesto. All in one day. Eula helps. When she naps, I keep going. I am unstoppable.

My full refrigerator says, "Finally, thank you."

In my recent blood test, I learn my hormones have stabilized— estrogen, progesterone, and testosterone are in balance. My adrenals, thyroid, and pelvic floor suddenly feel like almost no burden at all: only three elements now. I can't run, but I *can* move faster, and do a decent cartwheel. I'm fucking alive. Could it be this all might settle into a less front-and-center place, or even go away?

I cook and cook.

I can't stop making food and eating it.

I start to feel some version of unbroken.

~

After a hard late-summer rain, we drive country roads with the windows down.

"Mama, Mama?" Eula calls from the backseat.

"Yes, smooch?" I've begun to call her *smooch*, my smooch.

"What is that smell, Mama?" she asks, cranes her neck toward the outdoors, nose up, wants more of fresh.

"Rain on pavement, sweets, the best smell."

"What is it for?"

"What do you mean?"

"*What is it for?*"

"It lets us know rain came and rain might come again."

"Oh."

~

On the night of the blood moon, I lose about 85 percent of the hearing in my right ear. We are camping with friends and when I sit up after putting Eula to sleep, the world spins a notch, then so many notches, and my hands fly up to hold my head in place. I stand around a campfire and try to pay attention to conversation. My brain becomes a melon; strange underwater sounds swirl around and around and around somewhere within. I don't say anything to anyone. It will pass.

But it doesn't.

Standing makes me dizzy, sometimes, not always. This is my chance to act dignified in the moment of my body crumbling. I've grown, haven't I? I tell Chris and I am calm and un-triggered. I want him to say "I'm so sorry" but he can't authentically validate me yet. Our tension is still a sea monster under our sea. I don't push it. I let it be. This is all major progress for me. A few days later, Holcomb meets me in a parking lot at my request and pulls her otoscope out of her purse. As our girls play in the backseat, she investigates my ear.

No sign of infection.

"In fact," she says, "your ear canal is perfectly shaped. It's beautiful."

My options are (1) get an MRI, or (2) get bodywork and wait for it to shift. She asks me to keep her posted if anything changes or gets worse.

I make a decision. I will go to the hospital only if I fall over or my vision goes blurry, because then we're dealing with brain issue. No reason to overreact. Meanwhile, I have just started the Wilson's T3 protocol, under Holcomb's supervision. It's a naturopathic way to try to heal my thyroid and permanently elevate my body temperature to *normal*. It requires an increased-over-time dose of the thyroid hormone T3. It often doesn't work, but if it does, wow. Side effects: You might become irritable, tired, and/or aggressive. I don't know if I can afford to be any of those things, but I can't afford not to try the protocol. The ear issue happens on day two of the protocol. It's unrelated, but the timing compounds everything I am feeling. When I report the situation to an old healer friend, she says, "I'm so proud of you, it's a lot what you are doing, I'm so proud." I swallow and try not to cry into the phone. My head throbs in public. My parents host a dinner and I spend the evening unable to sit, walking around because the sound of conversation is like thousands of pinballs banging on my skull. I can't focus. The pressure behind my face hurts. Sometimes all I hear is a low *beep beep beep beep*. I don't complain. I am kind and pleasant. But this is a never-ending drive through an underground tunnel to nowhere.

So far, I haven't snapped.

Two weeks later, I still haven't snapped but nothing has changed. I make an appointment: acupuncture. It's an indulgence. With the exception of Holcomb and some Mayan abdominal massage, I've tried to go it alone without bodywork because how much money can a woman spend to try to heal? After it takes me over an hour to get Eula to sleep, Chris tells me my parents are coming over to eat dinner and watch the stars with us.

"I can't deal with that," I say, and two seconds later, they walk through the door. Wrapped up in her red down jacket and a furry baseball cap over her ears, my mother puts plates of food on our counter. My dad senses my mood and skulks back out to the dark. His reaction to me flashes me back to pregnancy. We all step outside. Cold. I explain I'm not feeling well. I try not to be mean, just quiet. They came over earlier and my mom swept and played with Eula while my father brushed the snow off my car.

They stay outdoors.

I go to bed. Up in our loft, under a heavy down blanket, I try to send my overwhelm out the window, toward the trees, where they can absorb it and send it off with the wind. "I love and accept myself completely," I repeat in whispers until the ache and regret in my throat subside. When Chris slips into bed, both the distance and closeness of his body set off a switch in me.

The sobs come fast.

"I'm trying so hard," I say.

He doesn't say anything. He can't understand my fear because it isn't his own. From the smallest oldest youngest most scared part of me comes the old question again: "What if I never heal?" He holds me and says back to me what I have said to him and others—this is my opportunity for a deeper healing.

The stars brighten out the window. Chris falls asleep and I curl up and watch them emerge from the dark. My head swells as more sobs usher out, as I consider that my family constellation has been exactly what I need, how both my body and rage have destroyed and healed me, again.

What am I not hearing now?

Why my ear?

As I fall asleep, my ear seems less plugged. In the morning, Eula will call out to me from below, "I had a good long sleep, Mama," and my memory will remind me of the previous night and the throb will inch back, until I am back, ear plugged, head thick, part of the process.

~

I make an appointment with rage. I've contained it for a few weeks now. As we make breakfast, the sun warms our earth and I ask for what I need.

"I need to go on a walk."

"Okay," Chris says in our white and wood kitchen. "Go for it." He doesn't ask why. He never asks why. I wish he would.

Eula, though, is curious. She puts her spoon back in her oatmeal and glances up at me. Why a walk now? Why is Mama going on a walk?

"Mama's feeling frustrated that her ear hurts," I explain, "so, I'm going to walk and stomp around." It sounds ridiculous saying it aloud but I am practicing a new language: less intellect, more body. Maybe Eula can grow into a human who knows how to articulate her feelings if she hears me try.

On the way up to the top of our hill, I start to whack at the air. These are gestures. I am warming up to the movement. It is also cold enough. We are on the descent through autumn toward winter. I know this is about my ear and everything before and now and after. I know I need to do this more often. I want to get ugly. I want to make myself a viper. I want to scream. We don't have many neighbors but sound here moves like wind, over hills, across meadows, and even in and out of the folds of mountain ranges. But here's where I have to go full throttle. I can't half bake this situation; otherwise it will lose power. My feet move faster. My energy builds.

Somewhere between trees and sky,
Somewhere between me and everywoman,
I become a weather system.
Body fumes.
Hands crash.
Face smashes into earth.
Yell.
Pound.

This is private. This is my mystery. One day I want to share it with others. One day I want witnesses. I'm not ready for that yet. On my way down the forested hill, with heat and sweat on my cheeks, I smell a sweetness on the breeze. Sniff. Sniff. Animal me. There are many ways to work an energy: build up, express, release.

This way is a good one.

I emerge from the trees and move toward our house.

I am a primordial human headed toward the home fire.

When I push open the front door, Eula beams up at me.

~

When Lauren arrives, our life clicks into fluorescent. She has come for a five-day visit. Eula wants to know what happened to her aunt's black jeans. Why are they broken? They are ripped, on purpose. She plays with Lauren's long necklaces. She watches how this woman with almond eyes moves. Later, when Lauren is gone, Eula will hike her pants up the way Lauren does. She is being introduced to punk chic humor emotion love.

"My sole purpose," Lauren says to Eula, "is to get you to say, *Yas, Queen,* and, *Speak, Woman,* by the time I leave." Eula smiles, unclear on the phrases but clear about a sense of inclusion. There is so much ease in our togetherness. We make faces in our cozy femaleness and I see in my daughter a flare for the dramatic. She has always gazed at herself in a mirror and practiced faces: happy, sad, shy, surprised, fierce.

Within twenty-four hours, we are picking animal cards. I get Otter: accept the feminine.

Within forty-eight hours, we are making dance videos. Lauren and I pump our arms and sway our hips as Eula run/dances between us squealing and yelling, *Speak, Woman! Speak, Woman!* I dance and don't pee on myself. It might be because I'm mid-cycle pre-ovulation, but I'll take it as hope.

Somewhere in all of this, I leave the house for two hours. At our first visit, an acupuncturist listened to my story and my pulses and offered this: my body has a lot of strong Chi to work with but is so deeply fatigued from the past three years it has forgotten it knows how to heal or that it can heal. Yes, I said, that sounds accurate. Now I tell her about my ear and the needles go where they need to in service of the unplug. We shall see. If it doesn't work, she will do some neuromuscular jaw and neck work next time. Okay, I say. I have to trust someone and she, with kind hands and deep voice, is an excellent person to trust.

With Lauren around, I haven't noticed my ear as much. It's present but doesn't assault me the same way. The days blend and we wonder aloud about Pat-Pat. What would she feel seeing us all here together? She *is* seeing us. In her physical disintegration, she must have softened. She must know that her great-granddaughter's un-shamed awareness of vulva, body, naked is a good thing. Maybe even the true sense of Catholic.

Pat-Pat must know so now, right?

Yas, Queen.

The night before Lauren leaves, we sit under the stars around a flickering pit fire. We may as well be the last humans on earth. Our one fire is surrounded by darkness everywhere. Crisp fall air. Eula snoozes inside. Chris has emerged. Where was he? Around. We each light a candle and speak a truth/want/prayer. I hear my man and remember his way with spirit is what drew me to him. He is so earnest. He doesn't falter. He almost cries, as he has done in many moments like this. I don't remember what any of us say, only what it feels like to be watching our blue candles melt into wood, fire, rock.

"There it is," one of us says.

It. The it of forever wanting.

Owls hoot nearby out into the blackness. I glance the stretch of silhouetted evergreen trees. They have witnessed so much recently.

Lauren gets on a plane and every plane Eula sees overhead for the next week is "Aunt Lolo going back to New York." We feel her absence. She has reminded me that joy is also a truth. Some bolt of energy has left with her and I feel responsible for ushering it up within my small family. It comes from history and lineage and shared blood. Shared blood, though, is broader to me now. It is woman-love-blood, any woman. I don't know what gender is anymore but do know what the presence of trusted women does to me. Whenever my mother leaves, I feel the same absence.

~

When I return from a full day of teaching, my mom lingers in the kitchen. She and Eula went on an adventure to town and then made a chicken vegetable soup. They also swept our concrete floor. With her hand down my shirt, nipple grabbed, Eula listens and nods and tells me about the day.

"We saw those big things, Mama, the big wings." She means the massive butterfly kite strung to the ceiling of the children's library.

"You did?" I say, and nuzzle her close to me.

"How's your ear?" my mom asks. I can tell by the softness in her voice she knows to tread with caution. Doesn't want to flip a switch in me. The ear has become a serious roadblock.

"It isn't much better," I say. "I don't know."

"Moll," she offers, "I think you need to slow down. Go back to basics. Food. Water. Exercise. And just focus on that, nothing else. You have so much going on. What if you start with feeding your body well, resting, going on long slow walks, that's it?"

For the first time, I hear this advice.

I hear it.

I hear her.

Two weeks later, the floodwaters open. After the acupuncturist works on releasing my jaw muscles, the sounds of the world start to integrate between my temples. In tandem, my pelvic floor shifts and now I pee on myself every day, often, without pressure, just by standing. Jaw. Pelvis. They are not separate. Another box of *Always*

Extra-Long Pads with Wings takes its place in the backseat of my car. I surprise myself by not overreacting. I hear the familiar crinkle of unwrapping a pad and try to trust that I won't always have to wear them.

Changes mean changes everywhere.

Life moves in cycles.

This is an opening.

The plug is gone, but my ear sounds come and go like tinnitus. When I'm tired or overwhelmed, it's loud, a built-in alarm system telling me to slow down. Even so, once it's better, I want to exercise. I hear my mom on the slow walks, but this creature also needs some amplification: weights, hot yoga, push-ups, core strength, rediscover my muscles. Because accountability helps, I tell Chris and sketch a weekly plan on a piece of scrap paper.

Yes, yes, yes.

Holcomb is on the verge of birth, so I go to an interim naturopath. The new doctor speaks plainly to me. She tells me there is only one way to heal my adrenals: rest, sleep as much as possible, eat well, create routine, and easy exercise. Go on walks and do only restorative yoga. Holcomb has said the same but I haven't been able to hear it until now. Really? I can't sweat? She doesn't want me to do any vigorous exercise. But what about losing the weight I want to lose? There is no way your body would lose excess weight right now with your adrenal and thyroid panel. It's in survival mode. My post-birth body is holding on tight. When I leave her office, part of my body shame evaporates.

Slow.

Simplify.

Old world.

I've been told that to heal I must not effort. My mom has had the answer all along. She would say I've had all the answers for her all along, even the uncomfortable ones. This is what we do—mothers and daughters. Her directive explodes everything I've known about how to be in the world.

It is so inconvenient.

It is also a way of personhood I've wanted to know for years.

~

What I learn: I learn what kind of woman I want to be. One who engages in periods of action and reflection, based on the seasons and her menstrual cycles. This woman is a sort of Amazon woman. She learns about her femaleness with her own hands and heart and voice. She learns about her femaleness in all relationships. There is no other way. Could there ever be? My mother has taken great care to remind me that I'm not and never have been *one big ball of rage*: "You are so many other dimensions, Molly." It's true. But rage is also a truth. In my devotedness to being a truth-teller, I wanted those around me to feel and know my rage. So few people actually show it. I would show it. I would crack my shadow open.

In the process, I became devoted to my rage. It was me and I was it. It was mine. *My* rage. This was dangerous. This ownership was aggravating it and making it worse. It was mine to manage but it wasn't actually mine. It wasn't me. It was an energy that needed to move through me: gray cloud, viper, tempest, hot fire. I imagine helping Eula through her own anger one day. It's okay, sweets, it's okay to feel it. It's passing through your body, what are you going to do with it? Keep it light, Janice had said to me about the incontinence. Don't focus on it. Don't make it yours. Do not identify with it. Do not clutch it to your chest. Thank it, though, this friend and other friends like sadness, for they are friends. They are the ones who led you to begin the emancipation of your feminine. Rage will cycle back to me again. I will meet it with a rhythm now. I will try to acknowledge, welcome, feel, and release it. My female body has shown me *how* to do so.

I will call it my postpartum awakening.

~

Eula catches a cold. We eat our breakfast together with the blue-black sky dark, and she says to us, "I'm gonna take my cold and throw it into the trees."

"You are?" I ask, laughing.

"You are?" Chris echoes, and squints at me.

"I sure am," she says.

She glances out the window at the swatch of green trees, her compadres who dance in wind and watch her while she goes about her day. You do it, girl, you send that hurt and illness back into Mama Earth. As we ready for her nap, she complains of her nose hurting, so raw from snot.

"I'm sick, Mama," she says.

"I know you are, sweets, it's hard to be sick," I say. The look on her face reminds me we all simply want to be seen when we are down. I lean over her bed, rub coconut oil on her nose, and she clutches my neck.

I say what I've been saying since she was born.

"I've got you, sweets, Mama's got you."

Later that night, we run through our usual bed prep. We peek out our wooden door to look for the moon and any shooting stars. As always, she asks me where, where, where are the shooting stars, Mama? I try to imagine how a child who has never seen one might envision a star shooting itself across the sky.

"It's got to be super dark to see them," I explain. I want her to grow into a person who knows that darkness is what illuminates stars.

They need each other.

Well before the next morning, before birds have woken up, Eula calls out for me. I climb down from the loft and crawl into her bed. We fall asleep holding each other's faces. When she wakes up, I pretend to be asleep. She sits up, arranges her animals, and then glides her hands over my bare chest like a manta ray.

"I've got you, Mama," she says, "I've got you. I love my mama." It becomes a chorus, a repetition of meaning and heart. When she stops, I open my eyes and smile up at her fresh face perched over mine.

"Mama," she says, "I was crying for you last night. I feel better after my crying."

"I'm so glad, smooch."

"You know what?" she asks.

"What?"

"My tears were falling like shooting stars."

~

At the end of October, we move through a strange sort of warmth. Wasps have infiltrated our house. They come in our open doors and hover at windowsills. Buzzing. Eula helps me trap them with a wine glass and release them back outside where "they will be happier." Because we can't bring her up to a loft with no railing, I sleep with her for the week she is sick.

We wake in the mornings to Chris who has been stung, again, by a wasp hidden in our bed. It happens enough times and he swells up enough times that I get my old EpiPen out so we have it on the ready.

"Oh, babe," I say.

"Oh, babe," Eula repeats as she strokes his cheek.

It doesn't escape me that so much of what I have done is sting him; we've stung each other. These days, in my evening prayers, I ask for help. I know to bring my requests (ideally) to Chris during pre-ovulation, after any hurt or anger has been moved through my body on my own. It may not always happen that way. I may need to say, "I'm upset/frustrated/angry and now I'm going to leave and take myself on a walk." Self-care. But how do I take extra care to say it the right way when I do bring it to him in full? I used to believe this question was a function of bending over backward unnecessarily for someone. Now I believe it's about dignity for self and others.

Here is the answer that comes:

You don't say anything unless you can be sure you have fed, watered, and moved your body well that day.

Wow. Okay.

A younger me would have said, "Fuck no. I say what I want to say no matter what. He can handle it." Now I know my mood *is* sculpted by how I engage with my body. Don't move it, I want to bash the walls in. Water it well and my thoughts flow like a peaceful creek. Create as clear a vessel as possible for your feelings so that you can identify what is authentic. Anger born of a sugar overdose may become destructive. But clear anger has an important message.

I hear this.

238

You, my dear, are the only one in charge.
This, my dear, is how we mature.

~

Frost covers the grass. As we shift into winter, I lie in bed at night and tell myself and the world I am willing to change. Are any of us *really* willing to change? If I want to change, I must again let go of the specialness of my story. My pain has made me so very special. Let me tell you about how I threw up for ten months of pregnancy, got transferred to the hospital then pushed for five hours, then peed all over myself for a few years, my thyroid gave out, I couldn't move, I couldn't walk with my daughter in the woods without smelling of urine, then my hormones, and then my adrenals, then my ear, and the rage overtook my body like an old lava deep in the earth, it could not be suppressed and my husband got it but didn't get it, and then . . .

Enough.

I want to refocus.

My mom teaches me how to make beef broth one cold late afternoon. I am trying to understand old ways. I am trying to slow down and name what kind of food, touch, and movement actually nourishes my body. We roast organic marrowbones and a gnarled-up joint with onion and carrots. The smell turns my stomach but I choose to like it. We stir a large pot as the broth boils.

"It has to cook for five hours," my mom explains.

"Okay, thanks, Mom," I say with an arm around her shoulder. "I'm excited to try it tomorrow." We are evolving our matrilineal lineage—women from other eras and landscapes and languages, women we don't know the names of and then Mary to Betta to Rosa to Ethel to Patricia to Mare to Molly to Eula. Our thread. We move shame, fear, and disassociation from the body out and out and out. The legacy morphs, lets go of colors, takes on new ones, releases limbs, grows new ones, breathes out rules, breathes in questions. This is always our gift to those who come after us. There are gifts from those who come after us too. Eula made a request when her elbow ripped an opening down my left side, my feminine side, from cervix to vagina. Wake up,

Mama. Wake up to yourself. What would we say to each other if we could gather?

It is now past ten o'clock at night. Everyone has gone to bed. I tend to the broth and arrange mason jars on the wooden counter. Our small dark house smells of the deepest part of an animal body. To be slow and full of a simple pleasure is the most feminine thing I've ever done.

I strain the broth into a separate bowl, then strain it again, then pour.

My mother saw in her daughter an urge to dwell on the body. Concerned this tendency would prevent her daughter from ease, she steered her as best she could away from such focus. Don't worry. Don't think about it. She couldn't know that the body was her daughter's teacher. Her stubborn daughter dug heels in further because she would not let anyone tell her how to be. Her daughter had to grow into a woman and then a mother before she began to understand what her mother meant all along.

This is how it often works, isn't it?

Honor thy mother; honor thyself.

At some point, I start doing a little broth-dance as I pour. Windows, silent trees, and Bru watch me. I am making broth. I am making broth for my family. I've got this. I've got this until my right hand pours scalding water all over my left hand and even still I've got this. I yank the freezer open and grab for a frozen item, pea bag too massive, what can I use, oh, chicken sausage. With a frozen package of meat on my hand, I continue to pour broth into mason jars.

So much meat for a woman who only started to eat meat six years ago.

So much body for a body.

There are moments we can see what once was and what now is.

Thank you, Mary, mother of mine. No turning back but to say thank you.

~

One afternoon, we tend to our home. I stuff clothes in the laundry. Eula runs around with her small red broom. My mother was surprised when she saw me teach my daughter how to clean. Why? It's an essential life skill. I now want to take care of the mundane and domestic. I would teach a son the same. If we can keep our rhythm at a clip today, I can actually deep clean the kitchen cabinets and scrub the shower floor.

"Mama, Mama, *look*."

She has plucked a swimsuit from a recent hand-me-down box.

Navy with ruffles along the top edge.

"Wow," I say with a stack of dish towels in my hands. "That looks fun."

"I want to put it on now, Mama."

Beyond our home, blustery weather has taken over. I glance out the window at a layer of frost over the world.

"You do?"

"Yeah, I sure do." It doesn't take her long to transform with some of my help. We drag a rug close to the woodstove and agree she'll be warm if she stays there. I continue to scurry around, but my eyes watch her—the way she strokes the straps, pulls at them, stares down at her new costume, the way an idea takes hold and suddenly blossoms on her face.

"Mama," she says, *"Mama*, you put your swimsuit on too!"

"Really?" I answer, about to yank out the mop.

"Yep, Mama, your stripey one," she says with an eager sparkle-smile, "we can do it together."

When I sit down in my swimsuit, goose bumps start to cover my legs. Huddled next to the fire, we grin at each other. I rub and warm my limbs up and realize there is nothing I would rather be doing than this—half naked on an indoor beach with my daughter on a winter's day. We are enjoying ourselves and we are radiant for it. Isn't this the true nature of the feminine? We point out the freckles we each have. Then Eula reaches over to my legs, strokes each one up and down with the touch of a feather.

"Mama, *look*, your legs are beauuuuu-tiful."

"Thanks, smooch. I know," I say, and I lean toward her, because I want her to believe I believe it's true, and maybe I'm starting to. "We love our legs, don't we? They do so much for us."

"They do," she says, and nods, an emphatic two-year-old, and then leaps up and darts toward the open pantry, where she has made a kitchen for herself on the bottom shelf. She grabs a small pot and wooden spoon and runs back over. The straps of her swimsuit slip from her shoulders.

"Oh-kay, I made some lemongrass sugar for us," she says, and thrusts a spoon at my mouth. How did she come up with that? Lemongrass likely from the essential oil I rub on my thyroid every morning.

"Mmmm, delicious, how did you make it?"

"Well, I poured it and make-d it, Mama."

And there we stay, for a few hours, under the gaze of our un-clean shed house, as we eat lemongrass sugar in our swimsuits and talk over the past week and stretch our long legs and make no effort to do anything but be together.

My daughter knows about pleasure.

I must also have known about pleasure once upon a time.

We know we are done when she tells me she's cold, even when curled in my lap. I am cold too. When we roll up, my body enters a world that has, it seems, over two decades later, turned upright.

~

Eula starts to see her future.

"When I am a woman," she says, and elaborates on how she will do the following: ride a horse, fast, fast, fast, go writing and teaching in town, ski down mountains all by herself, bleed like Mama with a string hanging from her vulva, read books with a lot of words, drink wine and eat chocolate because chocolate is strong, have long legs to run fast, jump rope, have lots of conversations because "I'm really into conversation" and climb high in trees.

Then she follows her bucket list with an important reminder.

"Mama, you know, I get to choose if I want to be a woman or a man."

"That is actually very true," I say.

"*Who* knows?" she laughs, and runs off.

I have done so much as a woman.

I have been a woman ready to abandon herself in the process of defending herself.

What kind of woman am I to be now?

She'll be a woman who listens when her body requests a slow-down.

She'll be a woman who plays with her own beauty.

She'll be a woman who climbs trees with her daughter.

That's what she'll be.

And the Moment to Expand

One week before conceiving our daughter, Chris and I walked twenty miles across a ridgeline. At the trailhead, we slept in our Jeep and woke at the darkest black of predawn. My eyes tracked ground, trees, and cliff as we began uphill. I saw shapes moving ahead of me. I stopped, clicked on my headlamp, what? Mountain goats. These white silent animals stared at us like ghosts as we stomped through their home. We reached the top, found an edge of the world. Pink had filtered through the dark.

Soon the sun would rise.

I had timed this walk with intention.

I wanted to do something symbolic with my body before becoming a vessel for someone else's body. That someone else had begun to float nearby. I could sense a presence, an approach.

There had been a hundred thousand moments where I thought, once I'm living there, once I'm doing that work, once January comes around, once Monday comes around, once sugar takes leave of my diet, once my ass is smaller, I will step into my beauty. I hated when other women talked that way because I did. My beauty had been a separate shell waiting to be inhabited. As each stage passed, I mourned it with a subterranean ache—well, I guess I'll never get to be a hot teenager, or flit unmoored through college, or power-dress it as a she-woman, or dye my hair blue, or feel my lungs pull me and a bike up a steep trail, or lounge around like a slender cat newlywed. Now would come motherhood.

Once you're a mother, you've crossed a threshold.

Order of operations.

I believed there would be no chance for recovery.

I needed to find my body, my beauty beforehand.

Let me define what I mean by *beautiful* because the word is as empty as it is holy.

It means nothing until it means everything.

Strong. Lean. Flushed. Awake. Exposed. Mystery. Graceful.

I'd found so much of that, but not all of it.

Chris thought the timing wasn't ideal for a child. We didn't have a house or place of our own to live, other than a yurt. We didn't have enough money. We were cranking with our self-employed work but not quite at a steady plateau. I told him to relax and get into it. We would both be right—the timing would be the worst *and* the best. I knew our child, a teacher, was coming for us.

Though I told him it could take months to get pregnant, we both knew it wouldn't.

"If anyone's fertile, it's you," he said. "It'll take one shot."

"We'll see."

We had waited to *try*, and part of this walk through dark, moonlight, and pink and eventual bright sun was about me willing myself to feel something. Time had run out, and now on this walk, carrying a backpack heavy with water bottles, I was trying to call beauty to me. I wore my shortest red shorts and spread my arms up to reach a cloudless sky. I couldn't distinguish the difference between pretending and being. If I had known that in a year, I would no longer be able to carry a heavy pack, maybe for the rest of my life, part of me would have died right there. But layers and layers of green brown mountains spoke something about myself to me, as they do to everyone.

The last half was downhill. My knees throbbed by the end.

So much downhill and no one expects the downhill.

It would take, as Chris knew, one shot.

On a bright summer evening, I moved over the top of him. Though wasps had stung him the day before, though his hands were swollen red, my mouth met his ear and I said, "Let's do it anyway." He didn't disagree.

Her cells multiplied as I continued living—camped on matted-down grass, drank bourbon in a small rural bar, wrote in my journal, prepared for my fall writing workshops, and danced at dusk with a friend visiting from Europe. I didn't know my daughter was beginning her life within me at that moment. I didn't feel it or sense it. I also had yet to consider that a woman's body grows humans (eyelashes, gallbladder, toes, femurs) without having to think about it.

Our female body is an art form.

No matter what messages it sends.

We took photos, my friend and I, before she headed home. We set up her advanced camera and ran ourselves out into the field above my future house to leap and jump and dance at dusk. Holler. Hoot. Spun, spun, spin. Our hips swung, our arms stretched up, up, up. Let's do it again. Okay. Then out of breath. Forty photos.

Shadows.

Such shadows—two women leap up and out against a dark blue sky.

I saw beauty in us, in me.

My shadow spoke: your daughter knows the drill and has grit. She comes from the divine and the divine requires both light and dark. Please remember, when you collapse, that I am your friend. No sore breasts. No food strangeness. I had not skipped my menses yet. No reason to take a pregnancy test yet, but I had noticed one thing: my pelvis had moved, deep incremental movements. Like tectonic plates, the flint of me opening to make a crater in the earth.

"I'm not sure I'm not pregnant," I told Chris.

Pregnancy would soon be full of sickness, but also of dreams of women lovemaking, me lovemaking with other faceless women, only women. Lesbian sex dreams the entire pregnancy. Woman, love yourself, love your mother, love the daughter growing with you, but start with love of self and all women. My body sounded a deep bellow, asked me to make it the sanctuary it was.

I could hear but not fully yet.
I had been born in winter on the ocean.
My mother had been born in summer on the plains.
My child would be born in spring in the mountains.

Mother

Every Sunday, Eula helps me water our houseplants with a mason jar. She knows the glass could break and holds it close to her body as she waddles across the concrete floor. Her small body leans over the palm, then the leafy fig. Water pools in the center. Stooped over at prayer, she goes about her task and hushes the plants.

"Ohhh, sweet little plant, I know you're thirsty. I'm here, I'm here."

These are my words. These are her words now.

She is two and a half years old.

She is a branch from my tree, her father's tree, and also her own tree altogether.

Ever since we've bathed together, ever since she's been capable of sitting up on her own, I've sung *I'm washing my body* and watched Eula watch me soap myself. I tried to adore my body even when I didn't want to. The example mattered to me. We are now in the flow of our evening routine. She is in the utility sink full of bubbles. I'm folding laundry next to her as she plays with her elephant, seal, and zebra. We are mother and daughter sharing alone moments together.

Then I hear her.

"I'm washing my body," she sings, "I'm washing my body," as she moves a washcloth up and down her leg, then her foot, belly, vulva, neck.

I feel her reverence.

I say nothing at all.

I pretend not to notice, until she catches my eye and grins. She knows. We know.

~

Mother can be a verb. It's orchestrated that our children teach us to mother ourselves. This is no inadequacy of our actual mothers. People must learn how to mother themselves. No one can support me but me. No one can support my organs but my own pelvic bowl. Interdependence within the mind/body, however, does not exclude interdependence with other humans. Do you know we are *made* to heal? My body had called out to me since the cold July day I was born on an island of eucalyptus trees.

I listened and didn't.

It called louder.

It had to call even louder.

This is the language of the body.

It wanted to be in conversation. My conversation with my body began as a girl on the ocean and soon became a dialogue with woundedness: for decades. My wound *was* me, made me clever and beyond my years and connected to realness in a world that seemed artificial. But when my body grew another body, it staged a protest. The wound had taken up too much space. We now needed that space for my underdeveloped parts (joy, sensual self, beauty)—they stood together and shouted, "What about us? We want to be heard!" And yet, the wound had been around for thousands of years. It had grown so large. I had to stroke it and spend most of my days with its myth and monologue. I had to introduce it to my friends and family. I had to thank it. At last, the wound had been heard. It was ready to take up less space.

I'm glad Eula saw me fall. One day, she will know her own falls are okay.

My daily question has become: How can I nourish myself? My slow-down has sped my healing up. Our modern world does not want anyone to slow down. You will miss out big time without the current herd. The herd moves fast across a varied landscape, creates community and exchange and learning and electric ideas. I want to be in the herd. But the herd has forgotten how to value the body.

I must unlearn that part.

Because here is the final verdict:

Healing doesn't happen in neat rows or columns. I will hold on to the possibility of miracles, that it can happen overnight for some people; but for me, now, it has been gradual. My incontinence has improved—non-issue the first fourteen days of my cycle. After ovulation, it appears and increases. So, I must continue my pelvic-floor exercises, sit as little as possible, squat, strengthen my core, and, then, see where it stands. If we have another baby, it might worsen before it gets better again, but I've intended a second birth and postpartum to be a healing one for me. I recognize that toning my pelvic bowl is a lifelong experience, just like keeping my legs or back strong and supple. If my incontinence isn't gone by my fortieth birthday, I will consider surgery. That is me softening. My adrenals will realign when I get out of fight-or-flight mode—as our routine settles, as Eula grows older and goes to school, as my sleep pattern goes back to normal. My thyroid is unclear. It's stable with medicine. I can try some naturopathic protocols to try to shift it, but my practice will have to be attention to food choices and self-care. The hypothyroidism is a state to monitor, not necessarily one that will go back to how it used to be. To prevent thyroid inflammation, I probably won't eat gluten ever again and I'm okay with that. And the ear, well, it's an expression of the whole package. It shows up when I'm overtired or overwhelmed. Otherwise, I don't notice it.

I don't see this as a failure.

My breaking has made me stronger and more agile of heart.

I'm no longer interested in whether I will, bar none, *heal*.

I'm interested in what a healed self now looks like to me.

It isn't going back to whatever my body was before. It's an integration of what was and what is, of choosing where to put my focus and light. Would I want to still be full of unexpressed rage and spewing it everywhere? No. Am I okay taking thyroid medicine every morning forever? Probably. Am I okay wearing pads to catch my urine for the rest of my life? No. Do I need to be able to leap and dance and run with my daughter? Absolutely.

There you go.

I didn't want to be a broken mother. I didn't want to be a broken woman. I didn't want to be a broken human. Who does? But to be broken isn't mutually exclusive from being whole. We're all broken.

It's okay.

It's okay.

These days, under dark covers before sleep, I ask my hands to beam and hold them over my adrenals, thyroid, pelvis, and ear.

"I'm here," I say.

My laboring woman is here too. She assures me she never went away. She's been with us all along—helping Eula and me, together and separate, go the deep. We are always in labor. Labor isn't toil. Labor is growth. Labor is where you meet your essential self. We are always birthing ourselves. She nods toward a woman who stands on a porch, legs sturdy as trees. Watch her, she says. You know her well, she repeats over and over. The woman holds her young daughter's hand. On her hip is space for another infant one day. She gazes across the grass toward a weather-beaten wooden gate. She passed through it to get here, where she is now: splinters, splinters often come in kindness. A breeze blows. Dirt pushes around. Stillness. Then hawks, the grasshoppers, then voles, then the earth. The woman turns to smile at me. She is radiant. She speaks the unspoken with care. Every day, she teaches herself again how to honor her taproot.

~

One evening, I sit next to our woodstove and listen to my husband. The candles from dinner still flicker and our pup sprawls nearby. Chris leans forward on the wood-and-canvas couch he recently built. He starts to speak in soft words.

We are reckoning.

"You wanted me to see you as the goddess during pregnancy and after, but you weren't the goddess, Molly. You were the opposite of that. And I could never tell you because there wasn't a safe space."

The bud at the base of my throat starts to bloom.

He never got to have a mood.

"And afterward," he says, "there are intense moments I've blocked out. I have my own trauma about what happened during that first year after Eula was born. I tried to help you but you wouldn't let me."

He's talking about me throwing laundry and "The Event" and probably others. So begins our shift into a more balanced exchange. My sad tears start to fall. I don't want to weep because I don't want to make this about me, but how can I not weep? Feel the feelings. Even when I wanted to hurt him, I never wanted to hurt him. He never judged. He retreated to protect himself.

"I'm so sorry," I cry. "I felt out of control and I didn't know how to share with you what I needed to share. I needed your attention, but I lashed out instead. I'm so sorry, babe."

He looks at the ground. I think he is receiving what I've said. For an instant, I consider adding how the goddess actually comes in all forms: both flower and death. All parts of her are divine. All parts of her have a message.

This is definitely not that moment, though.

Now I know about when and how—even when I forget.

Instead, I move toward him and we fall into each other's arms. His relief relieves me; his face is open and wide for the first time since my pregnancy. I think he has been heard. I won't apologize for my feelings or rage. Just like he doesn't need to apologize for his. He was mean too. But I am sorry for expecting him to rescue me. I am sorry for having pointed a significant portion of my anger at him. *My* unprocessed or misdirected anger hurts him and drains *my* brightness.

I want to move it through my body alone now.

It's okay to feel angry. It's not okay to attack people.

Who are we together? I have always been a woman who wanted to hug her husband while he was tromping somewhere in the mountains, trying to shoot an elk, an act he does not like but does for sustenance and to be with his brother and for the ritual of closing an animal's eyes, holding the heart, blessing over it. Once, when her menstrual cramps overcame her a few years into their togetherness, this man gave her a bath. He washed her body, unwrapped an o.b.

tampon, inserted it in her, and tucked her into bed. He was not scared of a woman's blood. He was so attentive—for a decade. When his attention waned at the exact moment she felt life had thrown her into a ditch, her claws started to grow. He focused on his own survival. His hands were numb because he was building their house and up at night with their daughter, doing his share, as his wife had requested, as they had agreed, and yet she wanted more.

She, this woman, is learning how to make requests.

She, this woman, is learning to see what is good.

Before bed that night, on the floor of our loft, I lie on my back and do pelvic-floor exercises. One of my writing students recently shared that she has been forever altered by her hard postpartum period. Years later and she doesn't think she can ever be the same. We pause and sigh. I hear her. The applesauce sours. The grenade blasts open. I don't think any of us are ever the same. I don't think Chris and I will ever be the same.

But that change was necessary.

I can, for once, listen and not bite.

I had to shatter part of myself.

He had to shatter part of himself.

When I zoom way out, I see the purpose of it all. It's good to apologize but we should probably also thank each other. Thank you for pushing me to the edge and then off the cliff. I needed to fall and meet my falling self.

As we wrap ourselves together, I feel his body release into slumber and gratefulness washes over me. He has been an integral part of us raising our daughter to be wise and proud of her body. My man can operate and see people separate from gender. He always has. When people asked if, as a man, he wanted a son, he responded by saying, "I want a human." Before my meetings or workshops, Eula watches me lean toward the mirror and put my cranberry lip stain on. She pulls at my leg and requests, "I want lipstick." I lean down, kiss her lips, and she licks them. Then, as if we are coworkers offering each other sandwiches, she asks Chris, as he pulls on work boots in the mudroom, "Papa, you want lipstick?" to which he says, "Sure," and she kisses my lipstick from her lips onto his and we are all, each one of us, set.

Later we will decide on a phrase to make passage across treacher-
ous waters, as they will come again, as they do.

Tell me more about that.

Tell me more about what you mean, what you feel, what you have
need to say. I actually invite you. Chris says I have never invited him.
He recognizes he hasn't invited me either. A few weeks later, we will
use the phrase in a tense moment and it will work.

Tell me more about that.

How would I retell our story for Eula? Your mama's fire grew so
hot it shone on all parts of the cave, parts they'd never seen before. All
at once, she and your papa could see all the clutter and dust in their
home. They cleaned it up. It was hard work, many days and many
nights, and their muscles grew tired and sometimes they gave up. But
they did it. From time to time, the dust blew in again. They learned
that dust always blows in. But now they each had a strong fire, and
they swept as they went and all was as it was.

Our love for each other is good animal love.

~

Here's what my body song could become: squat, sit as little as possible, untuck my tail, hang upside down, explore my core, use my
menstrual cycle to process emotions, dance around for most of my
day, nap, feed, and water myself well, talk to my pelvic bowl every
day, decorate myself, be among women, be among men, value gut
and pelvis as much as brain, lay hands on myself, move up and down
mountains, hug the center, feel into an earth-based, pre-language way
of being, respect the self, move the rage through and through and
through.

My song could sound effortful—do x, do y, do a, b, and g—but
it's only about one impulse: what my body longs for.

There has to be a body song.

We all have a body song.

My body is a safe and lovely place to be.

~

On an ordinary day during an ordinary week of an ordinary month, we eat bison burgers and salad as a family: my mother, father, husband, daughter, and me. Eula sits in her own chair on a big green box of old toys from my childhood. It's an impromptu dinner at the cabin, our familiar intergenerational living. I watch their faces and think of how we've all gone through a sort of earthquake together—the epicenter being me—and survived. My father pulls out the old photo albums because they crack him up. We kids look so European with tall socks and sandals.

"Eula, there's your mama," he says.

"There I am," I say.

She stares at a photo of me at her current age. On a lawn, my mother lounges back in her mauve swimsuit. There are other people nearby. She is laughing. I crawl naked around on her legs. My daughter puts her small finger on the photo and nods. We both have curls, big blue eyes—but we are wholly separate creatures. Somehow she seems to understand her mother was once a girl. That girl never expected this moment. That girl didn't know she would need to mother herself through many cycles until death.

We ready ourselves to go home: coat, hat, shoes, and goodbyes until tomorrow. The door opens and we step out of cozy and into the dark lead of night.

"It's so dark. Ooooooo, I love that," Eula says, and we walk past the guesthouse holding hands under a cold moonless sky. Papa and pup run and play out ahead of us, shadows among shadows, my man, my man-dog, my appreciation for them a deep thump in my chest. Trees watch. Eula keeps on and I say nothing but am impressed at her willingness to be so small on the ground in such a vast dark. When we reach the far out, near a stretch of cottonwoods and field, darkness consumes us. She asks me to pick her up, hurry, fast. Arms around my neck, she presses as close as she can to my torso.

"Mama, I don't love it anymore," she says.

"I understand that, sweets."

We look for shooting stars, flickers of light making their way to earth. Eula is scared of and drawn to them. Will they hurt her? No. Okay then. Her cheek warms my own as we walk down the long black driveway toward our home. Cottonwoods lean toward us and rustle. I have created every moment of my life to be a teacher for me. I hold to that early belief. How do I thank this child created from my body? She invited me into my female wound. I was both scared and drawn to the change.

There were so many small deaths.

But I have left nothing unfelt.

I want to welcome my dark and act with my light.

I have so many prayers for my daughter, for all daughters.

On the dark path, we watch watch watch for stars all the way home.

~

What I have learned: Every woman could catalogue the mystical convergence where her body meets her rage meets her shadow meets her facts meet her myth meets her joy meets her body again. There is no one narrative. The pelvis creates life. It must be true it can heal life as well.

I choose ceremony with my body.

I choose the healed ground.

Our female body, Eula, is both broken and whole. Does that sound heavy or hard? I want to repeat it to you. It is what I have learned. Do you hear me? We are broken and whole. We are whole and broken. They are both parts of a healed woman. We must tend to that language. There are no linear paths and we've known so by the asymmetry and symmetry of our body. Trust me. Do you hear me? Do you hear me as I call out to you now, and later, when I'm gone one day? Trust yourself. Trust that you will birth yourself over and over again and that's normal. Trust your ancestry beyond me, beyond bloodlines, all the way back to the sacred female in all of us humans.

She is, after all, the understory from which everything in our world grows.

She is, after all, the greatest story of all time.

~

Acknowledgments

Somehow this story has been waiting to tell itself for all thirty-eight years of my life. The process of putting it on paper created a healing of its own. Gail Hochman received this book with open arms and celebration. She asked critical questions to help sharpen my focus and wandered with me to make my words sing the right song. When Dan Smetanka told me I had written the book with my hair on fire, I knew that he *knew*. He has a remarkable ear for language and always knows when my prose is taking too many liberties for its own good. I thank him for his expert guidance, enthusiasm, and ability to make me laugh so hard my cheeks hurt.

Thank you to Megan Fishmann, Jennifer Abel Kovitz, and Sarah Baline for their tireless and smart work in spreading the news of this book. The whole team at Counterpoint Press and Catapult has been a dream team.

I wrote the first draft during a twelve-day residency at the Taft-Nicholson Environmental Humanities Center in the Centennial Valley of Montana. That time away from family and work responsibilities allowed the book to come to fruition. I will always be grateful for the quiet cabin and open stretches of dirt road. Every artist should be granted such an opportunity. Months earlier, on a summer day, I sat in the public library reading Isabelle Allende's *Paula* and happened upon my book structure; Brian Doyle's *Mink River* also introduced me to the possibility in a run-on sentence. These books gave me permission to experiment in the way I needed. For research, the following books gave me important insight: *Her Blood Is Gold* by Lara Owen, *The Healing Power of the Sacred Woman* by Christine Page, and *Wild Feminine* by Tami Lyn Kent. Books are living creatures. Thank you to those that draw us closer to the human heart.

My readers gave me confidence to know this story mattered. Thank you. Jennifer Gandin Le kept me real and generous on my page; Lauren Besser guarded my inner tiger and held the family story together; Hannah Miller helped me zoom out and zoom in; Courtney Martin validated and wondered and supported my efforts to start broader conversations; Jen Bloomer asked thoughtful questions and dialogued with me about the tricky stuff; Kelsey Sather ran over the manuscript with a fine-tooth comb and grew with me as we co-created Thunderhead Writers' Collective; Holcomb Darby gifted me with a grounded context and believed in this project from the very beginning.

Thank you to Mira Ptacin for her huge heart, inclusivity, and willingness to do anything to support the book, the collective uterus, and me. Laura Munson has been a friend, mentor, and fellow Montana writer soul sister. I thank her for her depth and presence.

Oh, the net that catches me is wide. Thank you to those who have influenced me during some part of this process: Janice Conti; Sophie Esser; Jen Marlow; Kate Seely; Kimberlee Auerbach Berlin; Dane Springmeyer; Sally Gepp; and Katinka Locascio, who introduced me to fertility awareness method, vulvas made of clay, breath, and the joys of New York City and continues to be one of my dearest go-to people. The Dabney women—Susan, Samantha, and Eliza—have shaped my girlhood and womanhood. I bow to Sam's ability to love and thrive under the hardest of circumstances. She is my clearest inspiration.

I remain ever thankful for my Bozeman clan of folks who continue to walk this parenthood and adulthood journey with me: Holcomb and Conor Darby, Louisa and Frank Carter (Frank was the #1 enthusiast for this book before having read it, and facilitated my time at Taft-Nicholson), Rebecca Fahrner and Mark Tumason, Sarah and Matt Skoglund, Cally and Dan Knapp, Geraldine Govaerts and Gregg Smith, Suzanne and Eric Bendick, Shasta Grenier, Sarah

Webb, Vanessa Skelton, Sara Wellington, Jaime June, Rae and Ryan Byrnes, and all the women of the Maternal Mental Health group who envisioned and created *Moms Like Me*, Anna Ourusoff, Stacey Tompkins, and Debby Greene.

Thank you to all the people in my writing workshops. You have taught me how to write and facilitate and be many layers of human.

Though a woman *does* the birthing, her support people are essential. Thank you to midwives Stacey Haugland and Kattie Jones and Dr. Luke Omohundro for shepherding Eula into this world safely. I am forever grateful for the decisions you each made during that twenty-four-hour period. Thank you to midwives April Mellito, Jazmin Price, and Kayla Wright and nurse Rae Byrnes for your support and care as our second babe grew and then made her way with ease into the water.

I often wonder what would have happened had I not crossed paths with Dr. Holcomb Johnston. We grew into pregnancy and motherhood together and she has navigated the dual roles of friend and doctor with such grace. I thank her for her devotion, humility, and intelligence. She got to the root of my health challenge right away. It prevented me years of climbing up the wrong tree. Every woman and man and child should have access to holistic care.

Thank you to my far-flung brothers, Peter and Alex, for growing me up and for being characters in my story. I miss you every day. My sister-in-law Valerie is all love and I am lucky to have her in my life. Rebecca, Charlie, Rachel, and Elena Besser read the passage about them and discussed it with openness and care. I thank them for always having my back. My cousin-friend-sister Lauren Besser is lifeblood for me. We live radically different lives and yet share a radical spirit.

My parents, Mary and Ken, lived this story with me. For five years, they have operated as a backbone for us—conversation, caring for grandkids, meals, and an upbeat presence just past the cottonwoods down a dirt driveway. They have taught me to believe anything is possible. I thank them for appreciating the truth-teller in me. My mom gave me her blessing before she knew what her role was in the book and, then knowing, gave it to me again. That says everything about her.

This is my story. It is also *our* story. Chris has always been my first reader. He has also, so far, been a main character in each of my books. Not once has he censored what I write about him or us. Above that, he created space for my writing, reminded me that my healing process was connected to my writing process, and continues to co-parent our kids with such love and play. He is our steady. We have journeyed through many weather systems together. I thank him for it all and for letting our story go public in the hope it helps other couples feel less alone.

My deepest thanks go to my girls, Eula and Bo, who set me on this path. You are both my healers. One of you cracked me open; the other has planted seeds in the crack. You are 4½ and 1 at the publication of this book. May it release you from my body story so you can live into your own. I wrote it for you and for all the girls and boys. Your generation is rewriting the script of how to be a person who expresses both the feminine and masculine. You already know how. I am eager to learn from you. I am so honored to be your mother.

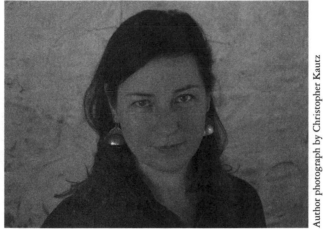

Author photograph by Christopher Kautz

ABOUT THE AUTHOR

MOLLY CARO MAY is the author of *The Map of Enough*. She received a writing fellowship at the Taft-Nicholson Environmental Humanities Center and her work has appeared in *Salon*, *The Hairpin*, *Orion*, and *Fourth Genre*. After living in six countries and eight U.S. states, she has now made a home in Montana, where she lives with her husband, two young daughters, and Great Dane mutt. Please visit her at www.mollycaromay.com.